A SANE DIET
FOR AN
INSANE WORLD

HESH GOLDSTEIN

Preface by

Patricia Bragg

ISBN: 0615779212

ISBN 13: 9780615779218

Library of Congress Control Number: 2013904415
CreateSpace Independent Publishing Platform
North Charleston, South Carolina

I dedicate this book to the millions of suffering people who are clueless about the healing effects of a sane diet.

What People Are Saying About A Sane Diet For An Insane World.

"This book is a "politically incorrect" masterpiece."

—Patrick McGean Director, Cellular
Matrix Study, Body Human Project est. 1999

"Hesh Goldstein is truly one of the few sane authors in an insane world, and his book is remarkable not only because it's incredibly well researched but also because it's delivered with a voice of courage and determination. While our sellout media broadcasts truly delusional health advice that only reflects the financial interests of its sponsors, Hesh brings you information that reflects the HUMAN interest of his readers. In a world of pharmaceutical profiteering, sick-care price gouging and the aggressive marketing of nutritionally-depleted foods, Hesh shatters the disinfo and lays out powerful, fundamental truths that can revolutionize any individual, any family, any community or even any nation that chooses to adopt them. You should read this book. You should LIVE by this book."

—Mike Adams, the Health Ranger,
editor of NaturalNews.com

"Hesh Goldstein's book is not for everyone. It is not for those timid souls for whom conformity to conventional thinking is more important than alignment with truth. I highly recommend it, though, for those who sense

that much of what we have been taught about nutrition serves corporate agendas rather than human and environmental health. A Sane Diet For An Insane World is a provocative read, guaranteed both to challenge and guide you. If you heed this book you will be grateful, because your mind will stretch and your body will thank you for the rest of your life."

--John Robbins, author *The Food Revolution, Diet For A New America, No Happy Cows,* and many other bestsellers.

"Hesh Goldstein has written a thought provoking, essential guide for people who want the truth about food. A Sane Diet For An Insane World is on the top of my recommended reading list."

—Kim Barnouin Co-Author of the New York Times Bestseller, Skinny Bitch

"Walk on the wild side with Hesh. Always entertaining and provocative, this is a book that will engage and challenge you. A must read!"

—Mike Anderson, Author of the Rave Diet and producer of the incredible video, Eating.

"Hesh has a real gem with this book. He has the ability to provide information in only a way he could—bold, unrelenting, and with a fearless delivery. This book will open your eyes and get you thinking about the next thing you put into your mouth and body. Without a doubt the content will raise some eyebrows. But Hesh loves people. This book is his gift to all of us. His knowledge as well as that of others whose wisdom he shares will show you a path to help you stick around longer and be healthy in the process. I highly recommend you read this book."

—Jonathan D'Alessio, Doctor of Oriental Medicine

"I first met Hesh Goldstein a couple of decades ago. Even though I worked in the Natural Foods Industry since 1970, I still thought Hesh was "radical"

in his ideas and delivery. But after a while there was no denying that what he was saying about nutrition was the truth. Throughout history, it has always been people like Hesh who make you stop and ask, "What is happening?" If you can get your personality and preconceived ideas out of the way, you cannot deny what Hesh is saying. For over 30 years he has been on the radio trying to turn people on to what is happening with our food supply. Terms that he uses to describe the medical establishment may seem extreme at first until you realize it is actually true. Hesh is like the first drops of rain before the monsoon. There is no denying that we are adrift in a sea of chemicals and petroleum based fertilizers that are poisoning our food and planet. If you want to make a difference in this world, read this book and live its wisdom."

—Damian Paul, Former president of The Hawaii
Organic Farmers Association & Farm Inspector

"Hesh Goldstein informs us, in his examples of "Tricks" from who he calls the "Pimps and Hookers," that those in charge do not always, in fact rarely, have our best interest at heart. We'd all be better off if, like Mr. Goldstein, we become proactive instead of reactive and speak out. As an example, in Hawaii so far we have resisted fluoridating our water supply. This is because of the likes of Mr. Goldstein who testified before the Hawaii State Legislature. He mocked the opposition by stating that if we approach health care like fluoridation of our drinking water, we may as well put Viagra in our water. I recommend Hesh's book for anyone who wants to be informed and make a difference. Hesh, keep up the good work!"

—Dr. Rex Niimoto, DC Pearlridge, Hawaii

"A compelling, shocking read." A Sane Diet for an Insane World calls into question information that you may have always taken for granted to be fact and forces you to examine your own choices."

—Christina O'Connor is the Assistant
Regional Editor for Midweek Magazine.

"Hesh Goldstein's book is a no-nonsense compendium of information to help humans make informed, common sense decisions about the foods they consume to maintain optimal health and the health of the planet. He discusses the many health implications of following an animal-based diet and makes a convincing case for switching to a plant-based diet. This is an ideal primer that includes plant-based recipes for anyone who asks, "Why should I change my diet?"

—Zel and Reuben Allen, publishers of *Vegetarians in Paradise*

Acknowledgments

With humble gratitude and endless appreciation, I would like to thank all those who have helped and supported me in my endeavor to bring this book to press. Without your kindness and support it would not have been possible.

"Doodles," my soul mate, who encourages me, supports me, tolerates me, helps me, captured my heart, and loves me despite my seldom conforming to the "rules" imposed by society, I don't know what I would do without you.

In all my years on the radio, I have been exposed to more health-related websites than Bayer has aspirin. As a result, I have selected my favorite articles from these many websites and have obtained permission from the website owners/editors to reproduce them. By doing so, I have compiled a "one-stop-shopping" place where everything relevant about the insanity of what most of the people in the west eat can be read. I never could have said it better than you have.

Dr. Fred Morgner, who became my instant "brother" when at five years old we met on the streets of Newark, NJ, I thank you for your incredible creativity and unique drawing style, that supplied the art work for the book's cover.

My deepest gratitude to the following individuals who have given me permission to use what they wrote:

Mike Adams, "The Health Ranger," of www.naturalnews.com.

Zel and Reuben Allen, of www.vegparadise.com.

Dr. Betty Martini of "Mission Possible World Health International" (www.mpwhi.com), the world's authority on the dangers of aspartame.

Dr. John McDougall, of www.drmcdougall.com.

John Robbins, of "Diet For A New America," "The Food Revolution," and more.

(For references within the articles re-printed with permission, please go to the applicable websites and view the original articles).

Mike Anderson, my friend, who wrote "The Rave Diet," offered at www.ravediet.com, having produced a DVD entitled, "Eating," which is by far the best I have ever seen on the subject, and a must view for everyone.

In addition to John Robbins, Mike Adams, Dr. McDougall, Mike Anderson, and Betty Martini who appeared as guests on my radio show, I humbly offer sincere thanks to the following who were guests on my radio show as well and who have enlightened me with their varying expertise.

In alphabetical order:

Dr. Neal Barnard   (Physicians' Committee For
                             Responsible Medicine)
Kim Barnouin   (Skinny Bitch)
Dr. Russell Blaylock   (The Blaylock Report)
Patricia Bragg   (Bragg Foods)
Chris Bryson   (The Fluoride Deception)
T. Colin Campbell   (The China Study)
Dr. Ronald Carlson   (Dentists Against Fluoride)
Dr. Paul Connett   (www.fluoridealert.org)
Dr. Bill Deagle   (www.nutrimedical.com)
Dr. Caldwell Esselstyn   (Prevent and Reverse Heart
                             Disease)
Randall Fitzgerald   (The 100 Year Lie)
Dr. Joel Fuhrman   (Eat To Live)
Dr. Michael Greger   (www.drgreger.org)
John Hammell   (www.nocodexgenocide.com)
Dr. Ruth Heidrich   (Race For Life)
Dr. Len Horowitz   (www.healthyworldstore.com)
Dr. David Kennedy   (On The Fluoride Myth)

Acknowledgments

Dr. John Kristofich	(Vegan Cardiologist)
Howard Lyman	(The Mad Cowboy)
Patrick McGean	(The Cellular Matrix Study)
Dr. Marion Nestle	(Food Politics)
Byron Richards	(Wellness Resources)
Dr. Terry Shintani	(The Eat More, Weigh Less Diet)
Jeffrey Smith	(Seeds of Deception)
Dr. Sherry Tenpenny	(Saying No To Vaccines)

Please go to my website - www.healthtalkhawaii.com - for a more comprehensive list of highly recommended websites and books.

Last but certainly not least, my heartfelt gratitude to Thomas Jefferson who created the Bill of Rights enabling me to take advantage of the First Amendment of the Constitution in exercising my right to Freedom of Speech. As a result, I have taken the liberty to give my educated opinions based on my years of research and study, since 1975, on numerous facts and figures written specifically for this book.

A Note From The Author

When I was a kid, if I were told that I'd be writing a book about diet and nutrition when I was older, I would've thought that whoever told me that was out of their mind. Living in Newark, New Jersey, my parents and I consumed anything and everything that had a face or a mother except for dead, rotting, pig bodies, although we did eat bacon (as if all the other decomposing flesh bodies were somehow miraculously clean). Going through high school and college it was no different. In fact, my dietary change did not come until I was in my 30's.

Just to put things in perspective, after I graduated from Weequahic High School, where I played football, swam and ran track, and before going to Seton Hall University, where I was Captain and MVP of our swimming team, I had a part-time job working for a butcher. (I mention the part about the athletics because that was my life. I lived to play ball and swim and like most kids my age, had no idea about how what I was eating would affect my life in the future). I was the delivery guy and occasionally had to go to the slaughterhouse to pick up products for the store. Needless to say, I had no consciousness nor awareness, as change never came then despite the horrors I witnessed on an almost daily basis. The employees would brag about how many cows they could kill in an hour and would laugh about how the cows would scream out in fear for their lives as if it were all normal to see these animals as a commodity that only served the purpose to die and be eaten.

After graduating with a degree in accounting from Seton Hall, I eventually got married and moved to a town called Livingston. Livingston was basically a yuppie community where everyone was judged by the neighborhood they lived in and their income. To say it was a "plastic" community would be an understatement.

Livingston and the shallowness finally got to me. I told my wife I was fed up and wanted to move. She made it clear she had to be near her friends and New York City. I finally got my act together and split for Colorado.

I was living with a lady in Aspen at the end of 1974, when one day she said, "Let's become vegetarians." I have no idea what possessed me to say it, but I said, "okay!" At that point I went to the freezer and took out about $100 worth of frozen, dead body parts and gave them to a welfare mother who lived behind us. Well, everything was great for about a week or so, and then the chick split with another guy.

So here I was, a vegetarian for a couple weeks, not really knowing what to do, how to cook, or basically how to prepare anything. For about a month, I was getting by on carrot sticks, celery sticks, and yogurt. Fortunately, when I went vegan in 1990, it was a simple and natural progression. Anyway, as I walked around Aspen town, I noticed a little vegetarian restaurant called, "The Little Kitchen."

Let me back up just a little bit. It was April of 1975, the snow was melting and the runoff of Ajax Mountain filled the streets full of knee-deep mud. Now, Aspen was great to ski in, but was a bummer to walk in when the snow was melting.

I was ready to call it quits and I needed a warmer place but for the time being I had to do something to tide me over having just lost my job with the Aspen Skiing Corporation. So, knowing that I was going to leave Aspen and basically a new vegetarian, I needed help. So, I cruised into the restaurant and told them my plight and asked them if they would teach me how to cook. I told them in return I would wash dishes and empty their trash. They then asked me what I did for a living and I told them I was an accountant.

The owner said to me, "Let's make a deal. You do our tax return and we'll feed you." So for the next couple of weeks I was doing their tax return, washing their dishes, emptying the trash, and learning as much as I could.

But, like I said, the mud was getting to me. So I picked up a travel book written by a guy named Foder. The name of the book was, "Hawaii."

Looking through the book I noticed that in Lahaina, on Maui, there was a little vegetarian restaurant called,"Mr. Natural's." I decided right then and there that I would go to Lahaina and work at "Mr. Natural's." To make a long story short, that's exactly what happened.

So, I'm working at "Mr. Natural's" and learning everything I can about my new dietary lifestyle - it was great. Every afternoon we would close for lunch at about 1 p.m. and go to the Sheraton Hotel in Ka'anapali and play volleyball, while somebody stayed behind to prepare dinner.

Since I was the new guy, and didn't really know how to cook, I never thought that I would be asked to stay behind to cook dinner. Well, one afternoon, that's exactly what happened; it was my turn. That posed a problem for me because I was at the point where I finally knew how to boil water.

I was desperate, clueless and basically up the creek without a paddle. Fortunately, there was a friend of mine sitting in the gazebo at the restaurant and I asked him if he knew how to cook. He said the only thing he knew how to cook was enchiladas. He said that his enchiladas were bean-less and dairy-less. I told him that I had no idea what an enchilada was or what he was talking about, but I needed him to show me because it was my turn to do the evening meal.

Well, the guys came back from playing volleyball and I'm asked what was for dinner. I told them enchiladas; the owner wasn't thrilled. I told him that mine were bean-less and dairy-less. When he tried the enchilada he said it was incredible. Being the humble guy that I was, I smiled and said, "You expected anything less?" It apparently was so good that it was the only item on the menu that we served twice a week. In fact, after about a week, we were selling five dozen every night we had them on the menu and people would walk around Lahaina broadcasting, 'enchilada's at "Natural's" tonight.' I never had to cook anything else.

A year later the restaurant closed, and somehow I gravitated to a little health food store in Wailuku. I never told anyone I was an accountant and basically relegated myself to being the truck driver. The guys who were running the health food store had friends in similar businesses and farms on many of the islands. I told them that if they could organize and form one company they could probably lock in the State. That's when they found out I was an accountant and "Down to Earth" was born. "Down to Earth" became the largest natural food store chain in the islands, and I was their Chief Financial Officer and co-manager of their biggest store for 13 years.

In 1981, I started to do a weekly radio show to try and expose people to a vegetarian diet and get them away from killing innocent creatures. I still do that show today. I pay for my own airtime and have no sponsors to not compromise my honesty. One bit of a hassle was the fact that I was forced to get a Masters Degree in Nutrition to shut up all the MD's that would call in asking for my credentials.

I left Down to Earth in 1989, got nationally certified as a sports injury massage therapist and started traveling the world with a bunch of guys that were making a martial arts movie. It was my job to take care of the stunt crew and the martial artists and teach a bit of my Wing Chun martial arts experience.

The interesting thing about this movie crew was that everyone involved was a vegetarian. When we travelled to other countries all the people that participated and helped us were vegetarians as well.

This bit of serendipity made me realize that being a vegetarian was not as abstract as I thought. It showed me that people worldwide embraced a vegetarian diet as being normal and not some weird cult thing. And even more interesting was the softness and compassion I experienced in everyone I encountered.

After doing that for about four years, I finally made it back to Honolulu and got a job as a massage therapist at the Honolulu Club, one of Hawaii's premier fitness clubs. It was there I met the love of my life who I have been with since 1998. She made me an offer I couldn't refuse. She said, "If you want to be with me you've got to stop working on naked women." So, I went back into accounting and was the Chief Financial Officer of a large construction company for many years.

The people I encountered at the Honolulu Club and construction company were the direct opposite of what I encountered with the movie guys. No one was vegetarian and all were hard. It was like being a fish out of water.

Going back to my Newark days when I was an infant, I had no idea what a "chicken" or "egg" or "fish" or "pig" or "cow" was. My parents thrust my dietary blueprint upon me as their parents thrust theirs upon them. It was by the grace of God that I was able to put things in their proper perspective and improve my health and elevate my consciousness.

The road that I started walking down in 1975 has finally led me to the point of writing this book. Hopefully, the information contained herein will be enlightening, motivating, and inspiring to encourage you to make different choices. Doing what we do out of conditioning is not always the best course to follow. I am hoping that by the grace of the many friends and personalities I have encountered along my path, you will have a better perspective of what road is the best road for you to travel on, not only for your health but your consciousness as well.

The other realization that I gained by being a vegetarian is that by adopting a vegetarian diet, aka a saturated-free diet, one truly becomes soft hearted. How can one escape being hard hearted, when one cares greatly for its pet dog or cat, but has no regard for the cow or the chicken or the fish or any other animal that one salivates over at the dinner table?

Everyone has a right to life!

Namaste!

Table of Contents

Preface

Dr. Paul C. Bragg, my father, was the founder of the American Health Movement and a worldwide Health Crusader. in 2012 we celebrated the 100th Anniversary of his Crusade and the founding of our Bragg Live Food Products Company.

My father lived in Hawaii for many years and was a health legend in its history of Health Pioneers who promoted healthful living throughout the Hawaiian Islands. Following in his footsteps, there are many who continue to spread the message of healthy living to the people of Hawaii. Each of these individuals has helped promote the message of healthy living in their own way. One of these unique individuals is Hesh Goldstein.

I have personally known Hesh, who lives in Honolulu Hawaii, for over 35 years. He is a true Health Crusader, Health Activist and a popular Health Radio Talk Show Host of *Health Talk.* I have been a guest on his dynamic, informative health show many times. He informs his listeners with vital health news that consumers need to know! He has a passion for sharing the latest information about GMOs, water quality, organic farming practices, and government regulations with regards to food production.

Hesh is not afraid to directly and aggressively address controversial, unhealthy issues and pulls no punches by letting the truth be known regarding conspiracies going on in the food industry. He goes after the industry when injustices made affect the health and wellbeing of the consumer. As a result, he often presents information on his radio show (as well as at public lectures), that will not be heard on food industry controlled TV, newspapers, and other media. He will not let the processed food industry and its commercial interests influence the viewpoints he shares.

Hesh walks his talk and is committed to following a healthy vegan diet and lifestyle. He keeps fit and teaches everyone he comes in contact with to do the same. I am pleased that he is now spreading his health message to an even wider audience through the introduction of his new book, <u>A Sane Diet For An Insane World</u>. It's an excellent read and a valuable resource for everyone who wants to learn how to achieve optimal health!

You'll find cutting-edge health information and knowledge that Hesh draws from the latest health research and from numerous health and nutrition experts. I highly recommend his book and encourage the reader to follow the teachings and principles it contains to achieve radiant health.

Dr. Patricia Bragg,
Pioneer Health Crusader, Health Educator, Author
Santa Barbara, California and Honolulu, Hawaii

Introduction

What would you do if you learned there was a concerted effort to keep you sick? And what would you do if you learned that the way it's accomplished is through the food that you eat? Would that upset you? Well, be prepared.

The best way for me to explain this is to put it in the vernacular of the street. We can look at the culprits as Pimps, Hookers, and Tricks.

If you were looking at it this way, who do you think the Pimps might be? The number one Pimp on my list is the pharmaceutical industry. Why is that? First of all they are all publicly traded companies and the first and foremost goal of a publicly traded company is to increase profits. The best way to increase profits is by increasing earnings per share. The best way to do that is to sell tons of the products you create and consumers buy.

The pharmaceutical industry, first and foremost, is in the business of selling drugs. In order to sell drugs, people have to be sick. They have to be sick either through natural causes or by inventing diseases. We'll get to the natural causes down the road.

Up until about eight years ago, we never heard of such a thing as "Restless Leg Syndrome." Before "Gastric Reflux Disease" took on such a fancy name, it was simply known as heartburn. These are just a couple of examples of how the pharmaceutical industry invents diseases to sell drugs. I wouldn't be surprised if they don't come up with a disease called "Refrigerator Door Syndrome." That label could be pinned on anyone who repeatedly opened the refrigerator door hoping something new would miraculously appear that wasn't there five minutes before. They could also come up with "Motivational Deficiency Disorder," which basically is a fancy label placed on anyone who was lazy. Another one could be "Consumption Deficit Anxiety Disorder", yet another label for someone being anxious because their neighbor has more toys than they do. I'm sure if you guys try, you could probably come up with some classic non-diseases of your own. And who knows, maybe you could market them to the pharmaceutical industry and get paid royalties for the rest of your life. (Mike Adams of naturalnews.com created the fictitious diseases).

The one thing they don't tell you when you take prescription drugs, is that because they're synthetic toxic chemicals, there is a really good chance that you will experience severe negative reactions to these drugs. To make matters worse, President George Bush made it so that you can't sue the pharmaceutical industry if you get sick or die. So basically, you're just subjected to taking their drugs and hoping for the best.

In the year 2007 or thereabouts, the Governor of Hawaii, Linda Lingle, spent $15 million of taxpayer money to stockpile the Tamiflu vaccine, which was supposed to ward off the bird flu pandemic that never came. The irony of this is that in 2009 it was proven that the Tamiflu vaccine was completely worthless and that it didn't work. (A groundbreaking article in 2009 published in the British Medical Journal accused Roche of misleading governments and physicians over the benefits of Tamiflu. Out of the ten studies cited by Roche, it turns out only two were ever published in science journals. And where is the original data from those two studies? LOST! The data disappeared. Files were discarded and the researcher of one of the studies said that he never saw the data and that Roche took care of all of it). The other scam was the H1N1 flu vaccine that was created to contain the swine flu pandemic. That one never materialized either but they sure sold a lot of vaccines. In Hawaii, because they were holding so many vaccines that never got used, they recommended that children, starting at six months, should get a second shot. Another nightmare is the Gardisil vaccine, which treats the papilloma virus. Not only are they giving it to young girls to prevent cervical cancer, now they want to give it to young boys as well. What they are not telling anybody is that this vaccine causes sterility. See what I mean about the pharmaceutical industry being a Pimp?

Other big Pimps on the planet are the large food companies. These guys are merciless. They don't care what they sell as long as they sell it and make a big profit. The best way to do that is to sell you food full of fat, sugar, and salt - the heavenly trio - to keep you hooked.

Most people are also hooked on a flesh-based diet. They are so addicted to this, due to conditioning, that it's hard for them to see reality. By the time an animal is slaughtered, that decomposing flesh doesn't make it to the supermarket for at least a week. Do you mean to tell me that after a week a dead body can remain as bright and rosy as you see it in the supermarket? And not only that, but you can walk into the supermarket and not be bowled over by the stench? So how do they take care of those problems? They use color enhancers and stink reducers. The ammonia kills the bacteria and the carbon monoxide keeps it pink and rosy and prevents it from smelling. Chicken is even worse. After the chickens are killed, if you'll pardon the expression, they are "cleansed" in a scalding, de-feathering bath full of pus, urine, doo-doo, and rot (the PETA website documents this). And the USDA says that if you cannot see the doo-doo through the clear wrap it is okay to sell.

When you buy food that is processed, you are buying something that is devoid of natural flavor and contains MSG, or a euphemism thereof, to give it its flavor. Did you ever wonder, when you go into a supermarket, how food could remain on the shelf for weeks without spoiling? Did you ever wonder why that is? It's because of all the preservatives that increase the shelf life that then increases the profit to avoid loss. With all that, you wonder if there is any concern whatsoever for your health?

In Hawaii, we have the rare distinction of being the Spam capitol of the world. We even have Spam festivals here. I have a friend who told me he was friends with the Hormel family children, who by the way are all vegetarians. They were forbidden to eat Spam. Hawaii also has another distinction - it is the colon cancer capitol of the world because of all the flesh that is regularly eaten in addition to Spam's "mystery meat." Some people will never learn.

Another outrageous Pimp is Monsanto. Monsanto says they will save the world with the food they produce - the genetically modified food they produce. What does that mean? It means that they take a food and make it impervious to whatever amount of their cash product "Round Up" they spray on it. In other words, they will spray the hell out of the food with their favorite pesticide to make sure that no weeds or bugs hinder the growth of their products. Just as a side note, in India they did an experiment. They went out into the woods and they hung normal food from one tree and genetically modified food from another tree. They came back a week later and found that the regular food was all eaten and the GMOs were untouched. It's not hard to realize that the animals are innately smarter than the people. We'll get more into GMO's later in the book.

Moving on to the Hookers, I guess the head of that group has to be the medical profession. With the best of intentions these guys go to medical school and wind up being subjected to curriculum that is funded by their Pimp, the pharmaceutical industry. When they graduate from medical school they come out with a "take-a-pill" or a "cut-it-out" mentality. To say that when a person graduates from medical school, they are nutritionally clueless is an understatement. When a doctor treats a patient for high blood pressure, high cholesterol, type-2 diabetes, arthritis, constipation, or whatever, it is always treated with drugs. When an oncologist treats a patient for cancer it is always with chemotherapy or radiation, depleting your immune system until it hits rock bottom. Nowhere, do they ever treat with nutrition.

Next, of course you have the mainstream media that will do everything to protect their advertising dollars. This, by the way, comes from pharmaceutical ads and ads from restaurants selling the foods that ensure you always see your doctor. Not only that, but the articles that appear somehow never favor plant-based diets or natural cures. Did you ever wonder why that is? It's all about money! The Hookers really give a damn about you being healthy. They only care about profit.

Then we have the government agencies. We have the FDA, affectionately known as the Fraud and Drug Administration; the CDC, affectionately known as the Centers For Deceit Control and Procrastination; the USDA, affectionately known as the US Department of A**holes, and the FTC, affectionately known as the Federal Treachery Commission. Why do I describe them as such? Because they do everything to protect big business and they do little to protect the people.

The FDA will do anything to further the profits of the drug industry. They have no qualms in shutting down companies dealing with natural

Introduction

remedies. In fact, the head guys at the FDA are former pharmaceutical executives. Right now, in the United States, the head of the Agriculture Department, Michael Taylor, affectionately known as "Monsanto Mike," used to be an attorney at Monsanto.

It is a known fact that cherry juice is a great remedy for arthritic pain. Yet, the cherry growers can't say that. If they do, the Fraud and Drug Administration will shut them down. Celestial Seasonings, the well-known tea company, made the mistake of saying that one of their teas was sweetened with Stevia, a natural herb. Well, the FDA wouldn't hear of that. So, they told them that if they didn't take Stevia, listed as a sweetener, off the label, they would shut them down—Pimps, Hookers and Tricks.

You all know that the CDC is a big pusher of fluoride. What a travesty that is, all by itself. But what you probably didn't know was that in their Morbidity and Mortality Weekly Report of August 17, 2001/ Volume 50/ Number RR-14, on Recommendations for Using Fluoride to Prevent and Control Dental Caries in the United States, in the third paragraph on page 4 it states," fluoride's predominant effect is post-eruptive and topical." This means it works on the surface of the tooth after the tooth has come into the mouth. Nowhere, anywhere, does it say you have to drink the poison. Even now, research is evolving and shows that the topical benefits are way less than they thought—Pimps, Hookers and Tricks.

The USDA is in bed with the dairy industry. The USDA protects the dairy industry as if it were a golden goose. Let me give you a good example: Back when Bill Clinton was the President, he hired Dr. Jocelyn Elders, a black woman, as his Surgeon General. Dr. Elders, when in office was going to make the announcement that blacks were 95% lactose intolerant, that Asians were 80% - 85% lactose intolerant, that Latinos were about 75% lactose intolerant and that Caucasians were 70% lactose intolerant. Dr. Elders only lasted 15 months. It's a classic case of a government agency protecting big business rather than the people.

Next on the Hooker list, we have the Public Health Officials. Boy oh boy, do they love to push vaccines full of mercury, thimerisol and toxic adjuvants. Autism anyone? Recently, an organization named "Autism Speaks" went public about trying to reverse autism. And they listed so many things that they were going to do. But somehow they failed to mention the vaccine connection. So I asked the Director of Autism Speaks, why that was so. I was told that vaccines do not contribute to autism. I then asked if the organization accepts donations from the pharmaceutical industry. The answer I received was, "not that much." Again, Pimps, Hookers and Tricks.

A child by six months old has received nine vaccines. By the time the child is seven years old it has received 47 vaccines. And by the time that person is 70 years old, they have received 160 vaccines. You really mean to tell me that there's no danger in this? In New Jersey and New York there are no exemptions to vaccines. They are trying to do the same thing in Hawaii.

Recently, in Hawaii, there was a hearing in which a bill was introduced to offer vegetarian and vegan meals in the public schools. The bill said that these meals "shall" be entered in the public schools. Two entities voted against this: The Board of Education and the Department of Health. When the wording of the bill was changed from "shall" to "should," meaning that now they had a choice to do it or not, these two entities voted in favor. Nothing like keeping kids sick and protecting the interests of the corporations.

I guess we also have to add the "shrinks" to the "Hooker" list. They are a group of jerks that invented "Attention Deficit Hyperactivity Disorder" as an excuse to put kids on drugs just because they might space-out in the classroom.

Then there are the dentists. Because they are hesitant to accept the low pay that Medicaid contributes, they advocate fluoride. What a convenient way to ease their guilt. In Alaska, where dentists seldom go, especially in the remote parts, there are people who are trained as DHATS (Dental Hygiene Attending Therapists). These people can basically do what dentists can do and are willing to go anywhere. Guess who opposes them? The dentists who refuse to go into the "boonies" to treat people.

I always love the organizations that are out there doing their work to find cures for various diseases. My favorite is the American Heart Association. These hypocrites have spent thirty years trying to find a cure for heart disease. Every year in Hawaii they have a Heart Ball to raise money to try to find a cure for heart disease. The cost to attend the Heart Ball is anywhere from $3500 - $5000 a plate. And the menu items: filet mignon, prime ribs, and veal. I guess they figure nobody would pay that much money for fried tofu, steamed vegetables, and brown rice.

Let's get back to Monsanto for a minute. We already talked about their GMO scam, but don't forget these are the people that gave us Agent Orange. We all know how wonderful this chemical is and the lasting effects of its exposure to our men who fought in Viet Nam. Recently, there was worldwide news that the bee colonies were collapsing. Why do you think that is? Because the bees have a hard time with the GMOs due to they're synthetic and unnatural. In addition to all of Monsanto's horrors, they are also involved with MSG and aspartame. Nothing like putting something out there that screws up your brain as well.

I've spent a lot of time talking on the Pimps and Hookers and not yet on the Tricks. If you want to know who the Tricks are, just look in the mirror. This is because it is our money they want at all costs.

Hopefully, at this point you have a clear indication as to why you have to take complete responsibility for your health. You have to understand one thing: adhering to a flesh-based diet will cause you to succumb to degenerative disease. And even though the animals have died so you can put them on your plate, they have the last laugh from the grave by giving you arthritis, heart disease, cancer, constipation, and type-2 diabetes, just for openers.

Basically, the only thing that can help you reverse your health or keep you in good health is proper nutrition. Poor nutrition will destroy people and good nutrition will save them.

Food plays an extremely important role in our health and has such a powerful impact on everything that matters in society. You all know that old saying; "You are what you eat." We are a diseased nation eating foods that we really should not eat.

The dead foods consumed in the western diet have been overcooked or microwaved, and processed foods have been bleached. Our diet lacks large quantities of fresh, living fruits and vegetables. It is a diet that avoids adequate water hydration and focuses on sugary beverages. It is a diet that includes large amounts of processed, homogenized, and pasteurized dairy products, which eliminate nutrients all together. What can we expect from something that has been cooked to 180 degrees Fahrenheit? Our diet is loaded with hundreds of different chemical food additives and preservatives. It is a diet consisting of conventionally grown pesticide-contaminated foods. It is a diet consisting of large quantities of unhealthy oils such as corn oil or soy oil or partially hydrogenated oils. It is a diet of heavily fried foods or foods cooked at such high temperatures that nutrients are destroyed while creating carcinogenic compounds. It is a diet comprised of refined sugar and enormous amounts of fat and salt. And all this is consumed by about 90% of the US population.

This diet, affectionately known as "the diet of death," adversely affects personal health, healthcare costs, and our children's ability to think clearly. This diet has a negative affect on corporate America because the workers poisoned by processed foods suffer from repeated sick days, the inability to focus, failure to learn, and failure to create new ideas. With their brains fueled by junk foods and with failed education giving them few options for earning an honest living, more people turn to crime. In time, the prisons become filled with people incarcerated for behavior that could have been at least partially prevented with proper nutrition. With disease rates skyrocketing, violent crime on the rise, education failures rampant, and healthcare costs bankrupting families, happiness hits an all-time low. As junk food consumption continues through multiple generations, the genetic integrity of the population declines. Then, because the population is dulled out because of all the junk foods consumed, economic productivity hits rock-bottom and employers shift jobs overseas where people seem to have much higher levels of productivity. To say this is a losing situation is a gross understatement.

Earlier in this section we talked about the pharmaceutical industry wanting to drug everyone and anyone to make a buck. But we really didn't talk about the problems that a medicated population invokes. Medicated drivers are no different than drunk drivers. Besides being hazardous while driving, this dullness also carries over to the workplace where medicated workers tend to make many more mistakes. You have people taking a medication to treat one disease that creates another disease, because of the adverse effects of the synthetic chemicals. And when those medications pass through the bodies of the consumers and eventually get dumped into the rivers and other waterways, they pollute the environment. And now, believe it or not, the FAA has relented and is allowing pilots to fly while on antidepressant drugs. Shades of Columbine!

This is a recipe for disaster: higher costs, lower productivity, increased rates of disease, decreased economic productivity, environmental destruction, and a dumbed-down population.

People in this country are addicted to fast foods and junk foods and live to eat rather than eat to live. And the insane diet coming from that premise has far more consequences than anyone can imagine.

In the pages to come, many of the things you have been conditioned to eat will be presented to you from a different perspective. It is my hope that by the time you finish this book you will have enough knowledge to make changes that will not only save and extend your life, but ones that will also enhance the quality of your life.

Let me leave you with one last thought: If there was a concerted effort to keep you sick so you could die early, assuming you would die before you reached age 67, who do you think might benefit? How about the government? And why? Doesn't Social Security kick in when you reach age 67? If you die before you reach that age, there is no danger of Social Security ever running out. That's because you won't be around to collect it at the age you are supposed to. Food for thought!

Aloha!

Part of this Introduction, in particular the last seven paragraphs, was written with the permission of Mike Adams. It is taken from his article, "Nutrition Can Save America," which appeared on www.naturalnews.com

Chapter 1

Saving The Planet? Not The Way The Media Hookers Tell It!

B ear in mind that the facts and figures you are about to read came from John Robbins, "The Food Revolution," which was written in 2001. Understand that things are not only much worse now, but all the quantities are greater.

Water required to produce 1 pound of California foods according to Soil and Water Specialists, University of California Agricultural Ex-tension, working with livestock farm advisors:

1 pound of lettuce 23 gallons
1 pound of tomatoes 23 gallons
1 pound of potatoes 24 gallons
1 pound of wheat 25 gallons
1 pound of carrots 33 gallons
1 pound of apples 49 gallons
1 pound of chicken 815 gallons
1 pound of beef 5,214 gallons

Let's put this water use into perspective:

If you shower each day for seven minutes, using a shower with a flow rate 2 gallons per minute, you are using 14 gallons per day (seven minutes x 2 gallons), or 98 gallons per week. Rounding that up to 100 gallons per week, and 52 weeks you would be using 5,200 gallons of water per year to take a daily shower.

Comparing 5,200 gallons of water used by taking a seven-minute shower every day for a year, to the 5,214 gallons of water it takes to produce a pound of beef, you can save more water by not eating four-quarter pounders then you will save by not showering for a year.

Your choice! Four-quarter pounders or a year's worth of showers!

Number of people whose food energy needs can be met by the food produced on 2.5 acres of land:

if the land is producing cabbage 23 people
if the land is producing potatoes 22 people
if the land is producing rice 19 people
if the lab is producing corn 17 people
if the land is producing wheat 15 people
if the land is producing chicken 2 people
if the land is producing milk 2 people
if the land is producing eggs 1 person
if the land is producing beef 1 person

"In a world where an estimated one in every six people goes hungry every day, the politics of meat consumption are increasingly heated, since meat production is an inefficient use of grain. The grain is used more efficiently when consumed by humans. Continued growth in meat output is dependent upon feeding grains to animals, creating competition for grain between affluent meat eaters and the world's poor."

- Worldwatch Institute

Where most Americans get their information about foods: Advertising!

Amount spent annually by Kellogg's to promote "Frosted Flakes: $ 40 million

Amount spent annually by the dairy industry on "milk mustache" ads: $190 million

Amount spent annually by McDonald's advertising its products: $800 million

Amount spent annually by the National Cancer Institute promoting fruits and vegetables: $1 million

---

"Although cattle grazing in the west has polluted more water, eroded more topsoil, killed more fish, displaced more wildlife, and destroyed more vegetation than any other land use, the American public pays ranchers to do it."

Ted Williams - environmental law author

"Genetically engineered crops were created not because they are productive but because they are patentable. Their economic value is oriented not toward helping subsistence farmers to feed themselves but toward feeding more livestock for the already overfed rich."

- Amory and Hunter Loving, founders
of the Rocky Mountain Institute

Diet And Cardiovascular Disease

Drop in heart disease risk for every 1% decrease in blood cholesterol:
3 - 4%
Blood cholesterol levels of vegetarians compared to non-vegetarians:
14% **lower**
Risk of death from heart disease for vegetarians compared to non-vegetarians: **half**

Blood cholesterol levels of vegans compared to non-vegetarians: 35%
lower
Intake of cholesterol for non-vegetarians: **300 to 500 mg per day**
Intake of cholesterol for lacto-ovo vegetarians: **150 - 300 mg per day**
Intake of cholesterol for vegans: **zero**

Average cholesterol level in the United States: 220
Average cholesterol level of U.S. vegetarians: 161
Average cholesterol level of U.S. vegans: 133

Percentage of adult daily value for saturated fat in one Double
Whopper with cheese: 130%
Percentage of an eight-year old child's daily value of saturated fat in
one Double Whopper with cheese: **more than 200%**

Time magazine reported that **cardiovascular disease is unknown in
regions where meat is scarce.**

Risk of dying during bypass surgery: 4.6% - 11.9%
Risk of permanent brain damage from bypass surgery: 15% - 44%
Recipients of bypass surgery for whom it prolongs life: 2%
Risk of death during angioplasty: 0.4% - 2.8%
Risk of major complication developing during angioplasty: 10%
Studies that have found that angioplasty prolongs life or prevents
heart attacks: **Zero**

Number of patients on Dr. Dean Ornish's vegan diet program that achieves reversal of atherosclerosis: **three out of every four.**
Average reduction in arterial blockage after five years on the Ornish program: 8%

Most current problem for which people go to doctors in the U.S.: **high blood pressure**
Ideal blood pressure without medication: 110/70 **or less**
Average blood pressure of vegetarians: 112/69
Average blood pressure of non-vegetarians: 122/80
Incidence of high blood pressure in meat eaters compared to vegetarians: **nearly triple**

Patients with high blood pressure who achieve substantial improvement after switching to a vegetarian diet: **30% - 70%**
Incidence of high blood pressure among senior citizens in the U.S.: **more than 50%**
Incidence of high blood pressure among senior citizens in countries eating traditional, low-fat, plant-based diets: **virtually none**

Diet And Cancer

Death rate from breast cancer in the United States: 22.4 per 100,000
Death rate from breast cancer in Japan: 6.3 per 100,000
Death rate from breast cancer in China: 4.6 per 100,000

(Now that Japan and China have adopted the Standard American Diet, breast cancer is skyrocketing).

Number of lives lost to colon cancer each year in the United States: 55,000
Risk of colon cancer for women who eat red meat daily compared to those who abstain: **250% greater**
Risk of colon cancer for people who eat red meat daily compared to those who either less than once a month; **38% greater**
Risk of colon cancer for people who eat poultry once a week compared to those who abstain: **55% greater**

Risk of colon cancer for people who eat poultry four times a week compared to those who abstain: 200% - 300% **greater**
Risk of colon cancer for people who eat beans, peas, or lentils at least twice a week compared to people who avoid these foods: 50% **lower**

Impacts on risk for colon cancer when diets are rich in the B-vitamin folic acid: 75% **lower**
Primary food sources of folic acid: **dark green leafy vegetables, beans, peas and lentils**

Most common cause of cancer mortality worldwide: **lung cancer**
Number of lives lost in the U.S. to lung cancer annually: 150,000
Impact on risk of lung cancer for people who frequently eat green, orange and yellow vegetables: 20% - 60% **reduction**
Impact on risk of lung cancer among people who consume a lot of apples, bananas and grapes: 40% **reduction**

Diet Costs the Economy More Than Smoking:

Annual medical costs in the United States directly attributable to smoking:
$65 billion
Annual medical costs in the United States directly attributable to meat consumption $60 - $120 billion

Most common cancer among American men: **prostate cancer**
Risk of prostate cancer for men who consume high amounts of dairy products: 70% **increase**
Risk of prostate cancer for men who consume soy milk daily: 70% **reduction**
Risk of prostate cancer for men whose intake of cruciferous vegetables (broccoli, Brussels sprouts, cabbage, cauliflower, collards, kale, mustard greens, turnips) is high: 41% **reduction**

Diet And Osteoporosis

Countries with the highest consumption of dairy products: **Finland, Sweden, United States, and England**
Countries with the highest rates of osteoporosis: **Finland, Sweden, United States, and England**

Daily calcium intake for African Americans: **more than 1,000 mg**
Daily calcium intake for black South Africans: **196 mg**
Hip fracture rate for African-Americans compared to black South Africans: **9 times greater**

Calcium intake in rural China: **one-half that of people in the United States**
Bone fracture rate in rural China: **one-fifth that of people in the United States**

Foods that when eaten produce the most calcium loss through urinary excretion: **animal protein and coffee**
Amount of calcium lost in the urine of a woman after eating a hamburger: **28 mg**
Amount of calcium lost in the urine of a woman after drinking a cup of coffee: **2 mg**
Average daily calcium intake of vegans: **437 mg - 1,100 mg**

Calcium absorption rates (according to the American Journal of Clinical Nutrition)

Brussels sprouts	63.8%
Mustard greens	57.8%
Broccoli	52.6%
Turnip greens	51.6%
Kale	32%
Cows milk	0%

Other Milk Facts:

Children with chronic constipation so intractable that it cannot be treated with laxatives who are cured by switching from cow's milk to soy milk: 44%
Lactose intolerance among people of Asian descent: 90% - 100%
Lactose intolerance among Native Americans: 95%
Lactose intolerance among people of African descent: 65% - 75%
Lactose intolerance among people of Italian descent: 65% - 70%
Lactose intolerance among people of Hispanic descent: 50% - 60%
Lactose intolerance among people of Caucasian descent: 10%

Average American's estimate when asked what percentage of adults worldwide do not drink milk: 1%
Actual number of adults worldwide who do not drink milk: 65%

Diet And Protein Needs

Protein in human mother's breast milk (as percentage of total calories): 5%
Human protein requirement (according to World Health Organization): 5% **of total calories**
Recommended protein requirement (according to Food and Nutrition Board of the National Academy of Sciences): 6% **of total calories**
Recommended protein requirement, including substantial added safety margin
(according to National Research Council): 8% **of total calories**

Primary disease linked to inadequate protein consumption: **kwashiorkor**
Number of cases of kwashiorkor in the United States: **virtually none**

Primary diseases linked to EXCESS protein consumption:
Osteoporosis and kidney disease
Number of cases of osteoporosis and kidney disease in the United States: **tens of millions**

Diet And Food-Borne Illness

"A report by the United States Department of Agriculture estimates that 89% of U.S. beef ground into patties contains traces of deadly E. coli strain."

—Reuters News Service

"Year after year the egg industry goes to congress to try to turn back public health improvements. Eggs remain at the top of the list that are causing food-borne outbreaks".

—Center for Science in the Public Interest

By contrast, 70% to 80% have been linked to diet and other behavioral factors".

—Karen Emmons, M.D., Dana-Farber Cancer Institute, Boston

"First it was E. coli and Salmonella poisoning, then the Mad Cow disease, and now the Hong Kong flu... what do these growing epidemics have in common? They all are transmitted to human consumers, through chickens and other animals raised in factory farms. And little wonder. In the filthy, crowded pens, harmless microorganisms mutate into virulent pathogens. Routine use of antibiotics ensures their resistance to life-saving drugs. It makes one nostalgic for the good old days when meat eating was associated only with heart disease, stroke, cancer, diabetes, and atherosclerosis."

—WorldWatch Journal

Primary source of E. coli 0157:H7 infections: **hamburgers and other forms of ground beef**
Potential consequences of ingestion of deadly E. coli bacteria in humans: **devastating illness with multiple organ failure and high death rate**
Long-term afflictions suffered by many survivors of E. coli poisoning: **epilepsy, blindness, lung damage, and kidney failure**

Leading cause of kidney failure in U. S. and Canadian children: **Hemolytic Uremic Syndrome**
Cases of Hemolytic Uremic Syndrome that are caused by E. coli poisoning: **85%**

Americans sickened from eating Salmonella-tainted eggs every year: **more than 650,000**
Americans killed from eating Salmonella-tainted eggs every year: **600**
Increase in Salmonella poisoning from raw or undercooked eggs between 1976 and 1986: **600%**

Annual Salmonella cases in Sweden: **800**
Annual Salmonella cases in the United States: **more than 1 million**

Leading cause of food-borne illness in the United States: **Campylobacter**
People in the United States who become ill with Campylobacter poisoning every day: **more than 5,000**
Annual Campylobacter-related fatalities in the United States: **more than 750**
Primary source of Campylobacter bacteria: **contaminated chicken flesh**
American chickens sufficiently contaminated with Campylobacter to cause illness: **70%**
American turkeys sufficiently contaminated with Campylobacter to cause illness: **90%**
Number of infected hens in three flocks screened for Campylobacter by University of Wisconsin researchers: **2,300**
Number of hens that were NOT infected with Campylobacter: **8**

Antibiotics produced in the U.S. annually: **25,000 tons**
Antibiotics administered to livestock in the U. S. annually: **10,000 tons**

Antibiotics allowed in U. S. milk: **80**
Antibiotics found in soymilk: **0**

Food Choices And The Environment

The contamination of the nation's waterways from pork manure run-off is extremely serious. Twenty tons of pork and other livestock manure are produced for every household in the country. We have strict laws governing the disposal of human waste, but the regulations are lax or often nonexistent for animal waste. A report by the United States Department of Agriculture estimates that 89% of U. S. beef ground into patties contains traces of the deadly E. coli strain. The impact of countless hooves and mouths over the years has done more to alter the type of vegetation and landforms of the west than all the water projects, strip mines, power plants, freeways, and subdivision developments combined.

Gallons of oil spilled by the Exxon Valdez: **12 million**
Gallons of waste spilled into the Neuse River in North Carolina on June 21, 1995, when a "lagoon" holding 8 acres of hog excrement burst: **25 million**
Fish killed as an immediate result of this: **10 - 14 million**
Fish whose breeding area was decimated by this disaster: **half of all the mid-east coast fish species**
Acres of coastal wetlands closed to shell fishing as a result: **364,000**

Amount of waste produced by North Carolina's 7 million factory-raised hogs, stored in reeking open cesspools, compared to the amount produced by the state's 6.5 million people: **4 to 1**
Relative concentration of pathogens in hog waste compared to human sewage: **10 to 100 times greater**

Number of poultry operations that are of sufficient size to be required to obtain a discharge permit under the Clean Water Act: **about 2,000**
Number that has actually done so: **39**

Number of the 22 largest animal factories in Missouri that are required to have valid operating discharge permits that actually have them: 2

Number one milk producing area in the U. S.: **California's Central Valley**
Amount of waste produced by the 1,600 dairies in California's Central Valley: **more than the entire human population of Texas**

Total number of water quality inspectors in California's Central Valley: 4
Cities that rely on California's Central Valley as a source of drinking water: **Los Angeles, San Diego, and most cities in between.**
Number of Californians whose drinking water is threatened by contamination from dairy manure: **20 million (65% of the state's population)**

Pathogen, stemming from dairy manure, that sickened 400,000 people and killed more than 100 people in Milwaukee in 1993: **Cryptosporidium**
Pathogen that Los Angeles metropolitan water district officials say is a constant threat to L. A. drinking water from Central Valley dairy waste: **Cryptosporidium**
Number of California beach closings due to water pollution in 1998: **5,285**

American feed for livestock takes so much energy to grow that it might as well be a petroleum by-product.

Calories of fossil fuel expended to produce 1 calorie of protein from soybeans: 2
Calories of fossil fuel expended to produce 1 calorie of protein from corn or wheat: 3
Calories of fossil fuel expended to produce 1 calorie of protein from beef: 78

Amount of greenhouse-warming carbon gas released by driving a typical American
car in one day: **3 kilograms**
Amount released by clearing and burning enough Costa Rican rainforest to produce
beef for one hamburger: **75 kilograms**

Length of time before the Costa Rican rainforest would be completely gone if it were cleared to produce enough beef for the people of Costa Rica to eat as much beef, per person, as the people of the United States: **1 year**

What a hamburger produced by clearing forests in India would cost if the real costs were included in the price rather than subsidized: **$200**

Most of the public lands in the west, and especially the southwest, are what you might call, 'cow burnt'. Almost anywhere and everywhere you go in the American west you find hordes of cows. They are a pest and a plague. They pollute our springs and rivers. They infest our canyons, valleys, meadows and forests. They graze off the native bluestems and grama and bunch grasses, leaving behind jungles of prickly pear. They trample down the native forbs and shrubs and cacti. They spread the exotic cheatgrass, the Russian thistle, and the crested wheat grass. Even when the cattle are not physically present, you see the dung and the flies and the mud and the dust and the general destruction. If you don't see it, you'll smell it.

The whole American west stinks of cattle.

World's mammalian species currently threatened with extinction: 25%
Leading cause of species in the tropical rain forests being threatened or eliminated: **livestock grazing**

Food Choices And Genetic Engineering

First and foremost, GMOs have been created simply and only to withstand a horrendous onslaught of Monsanto's cash crop, Roundup.

This technology is being promoted, in the face of concerns by respectable scientists and in the face of data to the contrary, by the very agencies that are supposed to be protecting human health and the environment. The bottom line is that we are confronted with the most powerful technology the world has ever known, and it is rapidly being deployed with almost no thought whatsoever to its consequences. Recently, "Monsanto Mike," a.k.a. Michael Taylor, the former Monsanto attorney, has been appointed as the head of the Department of Agriculture. Heaven help us.

Genetic engineering faces our society with problems unprecedented, not only in the history of science, but of life on earth. It places in human hands the capacity to redesign living organisms, the products of some 3 billion years of evolution, up to now. These living organisms have evolved very slowly and new forms have had plenty of time to settle in. Now whole proteins will be transposed overnight into wholly new "things," with consequences no one can foretell.

Going ahead in this direction may be not only unwise, but also dangerous. Potentially, they could breed new animal and plant diseases, new sources of cancer and untold epidemics.

Total global area planted in GMO crops, 1995: **negligible**
Total global area planted in GMO crops, 1996: **4 million acres**
Total global area planted in GMO crops, 1997: **27 million acres**
Total global area planted in GMO crops, 1998: **69 million acres**
Total global area planted in GMO crops, 1999: **99 million acres**
Total global area planted in GMO crops, 2009: **over 250 million acres**

Percentage of American cows injected with genetically engineered bovine growth hormone (rBGH): **about 25%.**

Why? **To increase milk production**
Insulin-like growth factor (IIGF-1) in rBGH milk vs. normal milk: **2-10 times as much**

Monsanto's suggestion to counter the bovine health problems related to rBGH use: **use more antibiotics.**

Chapter 2

Water, Water, Everywhere, And Hardly a Drop That's Fit To Drink (Opinion)

Would anyone in his or her right mind think of medicating the water supply to treat an illness or disease? You may think not, but this is precisely what has happened with water fluoridation. Fortunately, in Hawaii we have been successful in keeping fluoride out of our water supply except for the military bases, as all military bases are mandatorily fluoridated worldwide. I can understand that though, as one of fluoride's effects is to make one more docile and more apt to follow instructions.

The following is my testimony at one of our fluoride hearings:

I would like to pose some questions for you to consider:

What would you do if you suddenly found out that fluoride was not "safe and effective," but rather a carcinogenic, industrial waste?

What would you do if you learned that the sugar lobbyists' answer to cavity reduction is more fluoride rather than less sugar in the diet?

What would you think if you suddenly found out that fluoride does not stop tooth decay at all, but actually causes teeth to rot and crumble; and by the same mechanism, also causes osteoporosis?

What would you do if you found out that a myriad of research from other countries, showing that fluoride ingestion causes interference with brain development, had been purposely withheld from the people in the United States?

What would you do if you suddenly found out that fluoride inhibits antibody formation in the blood, depresses thyroid activity, promotes the development of bone cancer, causes premature aging of the human body, and is used in rat poison?

And after you found all this out, would it surprise you to learn that federal health agencies have known these facts for years, but have been controlled by the political interests of the nuclear arms, aluminum, and phosphate manufacturers to keep it a secret? Why would they do that? So that a toxic, industrial waste product could be passed off on the public as a nutrient with necessary health benefits. By doing this they also gain to the tune of $10 billion a year or more, going into the pockets of nuclear arms, aluminum and phosphate manufacturing industries, rather than spending that same amount of money to dispose of it properly as a toxic waste.

The public health officials and the big corporations with the vested interests portray those that oppose water fluoridation as "crackpots." From all the testimonies I have given against fluoridation in Hawaii, it has been interesting to me to see who comprises the "crackpots."

The "crackpots" are: accountants, engineers, chemistry professors, teachers, acupuncturists, dentists, the Union of Scientists at the EPA, and a host of others from all walks of life. We all come to give testimony armed with peer-reviewed scientific literature to back up what we have to say. Yet, the only thing that those who favor fluoridation come with is one mantra and one mantra only: that being, "It's safe and effective." How is it that they never have any scientific or peer-reviewed documentation to back that up? I think it would be interesting at this point, to take a look at some of the people who come with "credentials." In Hawaii, we have a Dental Chief at the Hawaii Department of Health named Dr. Mark Greer.

Back in the year 2000, Dr. Greer, on Hawaii Public Radio, made the statement that fluoride was safe because the toxicology tests done on it verify this. That sounds really great doesn't it? There's one problem though - only in 2006, by the National Research Council, was any independent, scientific, toxicology report done. The conclusion that the NRC came up with was that fluoride was toxic and dangerous to health, especially in quantities more than .8ppm.

After trying unsuccessfully several times to obtain a copy of the alleged toxicology report that Dr. Greer referred to, I had to go through the Attorney General's office to obtain the report under the Freedom of Information Act. It's funny that the several hundred-page report I received from Dr. Greer contained nothing about toxicology testing. I guess he never thought that I would read such a long, boring report. When you know that a person has missed his calling and should have been President of the Liar's Club, you leave nothing to chance.

So the question that arises is, why would a man in Dr. Greer's position deliberately lie? Does his insane desire to fluoridate the water supply take precedence over his integrity? Apparently and unbelievably it must!

There was another interesting situation that took place at Harvard University in late 2005 or early 2006. A doctoral student in the Dental School, Ms. Elise Bassin, submitted her doctoral thesis to the head of the Dental School, Dr. Chester Douglass. In her thesis, Ms. Bassin found a correlation between fluoride and bone cancer in adolescent boys. When Dr. Douglas released the thesis to the public, he omitted the part about bone cancer. About a year or so later the omission was discovered and Harvard conducted an investigation. Dr. Douglas was exonerated. We wonder if the fact that he donated $1 million to Harvard, while the investigation was going on, and that he was on the payroll of the Colgate/Palmolive Company, had anything to do with it?

In that same National Research Council report it was concluded that fluoridated water should not be used in infant formula due to the danger of neurological damage. It was also concluded that kidney patients, diabetics, seniors, and outdoor workers were susceptible populations and especially vulnerable to harm from fluoride ingestion. Yet many dentists and many of the States' Dental Associations, as well as our public health officials, neglected to pass on that message for quite some time. Do you think it might be hard for some people to admit they may be wrong about something?

Before organized dentistry became fluoride fixated and before fluoride was mandated, a 1950 Connecticut study clearly linked more fruit and vegetable consumption and less sugar consumption to fewer cavities. Did you know that a 20-ounce bottle of soda contains 14 teaspoons of sugar and a 7-11 "Big Gulp" contains 56 teaspoons of sugar? If there were any more than that the sugar would be too heavy and settle to the bottom. But, I guess the dentists' answer to that situation would be that if the soda were made with fluoridated water, cavities could be prevented. Riiiight!

After sixty years of water fluoridation, reaching two thirds of Americans via public water supplies, and virtually 100% of the food supply and fluoridated dental products (ensuring a multibillion-dollar international business) up to one half of US schoolchildren sport fluoride overdose symptoms. These systems show up as dental fluorosis - which is white, yellow or brown, and sometimes pitted, teeth.

Tooth decay is still a national epidemic, especially among the low-income people who cannot find dentists willing or able to fix their rotting teeth. And why are the dentists not willing or able to treat these low-income people? Because the amount that Medicaid pays is too low for them to accept.

There's another situation that needs to be brought to light regarding a noted and well-established neuro-toxicologist, Dr. Phyllis Mullenix. Dr. Mullenix's research proves that fluoride is a neurotoxin affecting the central nervous system. When she published her work in 1995, it was not only dismissed, but it also ended her career. What is ironic is that one of her mentors, Dr. Harold Hodge, who served as the chief toxicologist for the Manhattan Project, a.k.a. the Atomic Energy Commission, was instrumental in selling fluoride to the public. As Dr. Mullenix's work progressed, and she reported her findings to Hodge, he shrugged them off. It wasn't until much later that Dr. Mullenix learned that Hodge had conducted his own research fifty years earlier, and had first discovered the connection between fluoride and its ill effects on the central nervous system.

Many of the early opponents of water fluoridation recognized that fluoride was a critical component in uranium and aluminum production, and necessary in the making of the "bomb." Common sense told them that adding the waste product of a chemical that can cut through steel is bound to have some adverse health effects in the body. Despite their best efforts, a massive public relations campaign was waged and won, and fluoride was shoved into public drinking water supplies and into dental curriculums - a neat and tidy solution to the expensive problem of what to do with toxic waste. And, much of the research supporting fluoridation came from industry-funded studies. How objective can you get?

The National Research Council advises that more studies are required on fluoride's effects. These effects cover reasoning ability, endocrine functions, immune deficiencies, fertility, gastric response, bladder cancer, kidney and liver enzyme functions, arthritis-like conditions, and more.

Peer-reviewed studies already link fluoride to cancer, genetic defects, IQ deficiencies, thyroid dysfunction, gum disease, kidney, tooth and bone damage, and symptoms characteristic of Alzheimer's disease. In fact, medical reports from India had indicated that arthritic type symptoms have disappeared when test subjects stopped using fluoridated toothpaste.

So why do the dental associations and the public health officials still cling to the idea that fluoridation is good? Denial? Dental school indoctrination? Embarrassment that they have been wrong all along? Possible liability associated with all the deleterious health effects people have suffered from fluoride being thrust upon them against their will? I guess that it's more convenient to carry on with the idea that fluoridation is beneficial than to lose face!

I would like to offer some information that I'm sure you will find very interesting and worth some thought. The CDC, in their Morbidity and Mortality weekly report on "Recommendations for Using Fluoride to Prevent and Control Dental Caries in the United States," August 17, 2001/ Vol. 50/ No. RR-14, on page 4, fourth paragraph, it says: "The laboratory and epidemiologic research that has led to the better understanding of how fluoride prevents dental caries indicates that fluoride's predominant effect is post-eruptive (after the tooth has come into the mouth) and topical (on the surface of the tooth) and that the effects depends on fluoride being in the right amount in the right place at the right time." Nowhere does it say you have to drink it.

Consider this: under the Pure Water Drinking Act, it is illegal to dump fluoride in the lakes, streams, and oceans. But, for some weird reason, it is deemed okay for fluoride to enter these same bodies of water if it passes through a water faucet and a person's body first.

How is that for theater of the absurd?

References: Dr. Paul Connett's website, www.fluoridealert.org, will give you so much information that you will never want to ever drink this crap again. Maybe it will inspire you to become a "crackpot" and fight to get it out of your water supply.

Chapter 3

Why Say No To GMOs

First, the less obvious:

Did you know ... if seeds from a GMO field blow over to a non-GMO field the non-GMO farmer can be sued for theft?

Did you know ... normally, a farmer holds seeds to be used for the next season. But Monsanto, who must be hurting for money, makes GMO farmers buy new seeds every year?

Did you know ... why GMO foods are not labeled is because Monsanto paid off whoever to make sure that GMO foods do NOT get labeled as such? Do you think they did that because they knew that no one would buy them if they were labeled?

Did you know ... why GMO foods are so readily accepted by the "Fraud and Drug Administration?" I wonder if Monsanto's former top executives holding key positions in the FDA have anything to do with that?

Did you know ... since 1996 Americans have been eating genetically modified ingredients in most processed foods?

Did you know ... genetically modified plants, such as soybean, corn, cottonseed, canola (what's a canola?) and now sugar beets and alfalfa have had foreign genes forced into their DNA and the inserted genes come from bacteria and viruses that have never been in the human food supply?

Did you know ... GMOs have been linked to thousands of toxic and allergic reactions, thousands of sick, sterile and dead livestock, and damage to virtually every organ and system studied in lab animals?

Did you know ... in India an experiment was performed. People went out to the "boonies." They hung GMO foods from one tree and non-GMO foods from another tree. A week later they came back and found that all the non-GMO foods were eaten and all of the GMO foods were untouched. It seems that the animals have more innate intelligence than the people.

Did you know ... the Fraud and drug Administration has approved the use of 2-4-D, the active ingredient in Agent Orange, to be sprayed on the corn fields in the U.S.?

Did you know ... Agent Orange decimated the jungle in in Viet Nam, gave many of our armed forces that were exposed to it, cancer, and left the Vietnamese with an enormous array of birth defects in their children? Despite all of this, Monsanto says that 2-4-D is safe to eat and GMOs need not be labeled.

In 1992, the "Fraud and Drug Administration" claimed that they had no information showing that genetically modified foods were substantially different from conventionally grown foods and therefore were safe to eat. But, internal memos made public by a lawsuit revealed that political appointees under orders from the White House to promote GMOs staged their position. FDA scientists, on the other hand, warned that GMOs could create unpredictable, genetically hard-to-detect side effects including allergies, toxins, new diseases, and nutritional problems. They urged long-term safety studies, but were ignored. Why? It's because the "Fraud and Drug Administration" does not require any safety evaluations for GMOs. Instead, biotech companies, which have been found guilty of hiding the toxic effects of their chemical products, are now in charge of determining whether their GMO foods are safe. The FDA official in charge of creating this policy was Michael Taylor, Monsanto's former attorney and later its vice-president.

Although these biotech companies participate in a voluntary consultation process with the FDA, it is a meaningless exercise. The summaries of the superficial research they submit cannot identify most of the health risks of GMOs.

In contrast to the statements of biotech advocates, FDA scientists and others affirm that genetic modification is not just an extension of the conventional breeding techniques that have been used by farmers for lifetimes. Genetic engineering transfers genes across natural species barriers, using imprecise laboratory techniques that bear no resemblance to natural breeding. Furthermore, the technology is based on outdated concepts of how genes and cells work.

Gene insertion is done either by shooting genes from a "gene gun" into a plate of cells, or by using bacteria to invade the cell with foreign DNA. The altered cell is then cloned into a plant. These processes create massive collateral damage, causing mutations in hundreds or thousands of locations throughout the plant's DNA. Natural genes can be deleted or permanently turned on or off, and hundreds may change their levels of expression. In addition, the inserted gene is often rearranged, may transfer from the food into our body's cells or into the DNA of bacteria inside us, and the GMO protein produced by the gene may have unintended properties or effects.

The primary reason companies genetically engineer plants are to make them tolerant to their brand of herbicide and pesticide. The four major genetically modified plants, soy, corn, canola, and cotton and now, sugar beets and alfalfa are designed to survive an otherwise deadly dose of weed killer. These crops have much higher residues of toxic herbicides. Basically, Monsanto created GMOs to withstand enormous amounts of their "cash crop," Roundup *(see end of article for some interesting bits about Roundup).

The second GMO trait is a built-in pesticide. A gene from the soil bacterium called Bt (Bacillus thuringiensis) is inserted into cotton and corn DNA, where it secretes the insect-killing Bt-toxin in every cell. About 19% of genetically modified crops produce their own pesticide. Another 13% produce a pesticide and are herbicide/pesticide tolerant.

Also, small amounts of zucchini, and yellow crookneck squash as well as Hawaiian papaya are engineered to resist plant viruses. In fact, virtually all Hawaiian papaya is genetically modified.

Now, let's take a look at some of the evidence of harm from GMOs:

Soy allergies skyrocketed by 50% in the UK soon after GMO soy was introduced.

A human subject showed a skin prick allergic-type reaction to GMO soy, but not to natural soy.

The level of one known soy allergen is as much as seven-times higher in cooked genetically modified soy compared to non-genetically modified soy.

Genetically modified soy also contains an unexpected allergen-type protein not found in natural soy. The biotech industry claims that the Bt-toxin found in corn and cotton is harmless to humans and mammals because "the natural bacteria version has been used as a spray by farmers for years." In reality, hundreds of people exposed to Bt spray had allergic-type symptoms and mice fed Bt had powerful immune responses and damaged intestines. Bt in genetically modified crops is designed to be more toxic than the natural spray and is thousands of times more concentrated.

Hundreds of laborers in India report allergic reactions just from handling Bt cotton and their symptoms are identical to those exposed to Bt spray.

No tests can guarantee that a GMO will not cause allergies. Although the World Health Organization recommends a protein screening protocol, the genetically modified soy, corn, and papaya in our food supply fail these tests because they have properties of known allergens.

If proteins digest slowly, there is more time for allergic reactions. Because genetically modified soy reduces digestive enzymes in mice, it may slow protein digestion and promote allergies to many foods.

Mice not only reacted to Bt-toxin, they had immune responses to formerly harmless compounds.

Similarly, a mouse test indicated that people eating genetically modified peas could develop allergies to the peas and to a range of other foods. The peas had already passed all allergy tests normally used to get GMOs on the market. It took this advanced mouse test, which was never used on the GMOs we eat, to discover that the peas could be deadly.

Rats fed genetically modified potatoes had smaller, partially atrophied livers.

The livers of rats fed genetically modified canola were 12-16% heavier.

Genetically modified soy altered mouse liver cells in ways that suggest a toxic insult. The changes reversed after their diet switched to non-genetically modified soy.

More than half the offspring of mother rats fed genetically modified soy, died within three weeks.

Male rats and mice fed genetically modified soy showed changes in their testicles; the mice had altered young sperm cells.

The DNA of mouse embryos whose parents ate genetically modified soy functioned differently than those whose parents ate non- genetically modified soy.

When sheep grazed on Bt cotton plants after harvest, within a week one in four died.

Farmers in Europe and Asia say that cows, water buffaloes, chickens, and horses died from eating Bt corn varieties.

About two-dozen US farmers report that Bt corn varieties caused widespread sterility in pigs and cows.

Filipinos in at least five villages fell sick when a nearby Bt corn variety was pollinating.

The stomach lining of rats fed genetically modified potatoes showed excessive cell growth, a condition that may be a precursor to cancer. Rats also had damaged organs and immune systems.

Unlike safety evaluations for drugs, there are no human clinical trials of genetically modified foods. The only published human feeding experiment verified that genetic material inserted into genetically modified soy transfers into the DNA of intestinal bacteria and continues to function. This means that long after we stop eating genetically modified foods, we may still have their genetically modified proteins continuously working inside us.

If the antibiotic gene inserted into most genetically modified crops were to transfer to us, it could create super diseases resistant to antibiotics.

If the gene that creates Bt-toxin in genetically modified corn were to transfer to us, it might turn our intestinal flora into living pesticide factories.

Animal studies show that DNA in food can travel into organs throughout the body—even into fetuses.

Morgellon's Disease, which is experienced as bugs crawling under your skin, is linked to GMOs.

In the 1980's, a contaminated brand of a food supplement called L-tryptophan killed 100 Americans and caused sickness and disability in another 5,000 - 10,000 people. The source of the contaminants was almost certainly the genetic engineering process used in its production. The disease took years to find and was almost overlooked. It was only because the symptoms were unique, acute, and fast acting. If all three characteristics were not in place, the deadly genetically modified supplement might never have been identified or removed.

If GMO foods on the market are causing common diseases or if their effects appear only after long-term exposure, we may not be able to identify the source of the problem for decades, if at all. There is no monitoring of GMO-related problems and no long-term animal studies underway. Heavily invested biotech corporations are gambling away the health of our world for profit.

This was confirmed by a study done in 2013 by two scientists – Anthony Samsel and Dr. Stephannie Semff of MIT. Their report entitled, Glyphosate's Suppression of Cytochrome P450 Enzymes and Amino Acid Biosynthesis by the Gut Microbiome: Pathways to Modern Diseases.

They reported that the effects of glyphosate, the active ingredient in Monsanto's Roundup Ready herbicide, are insidious because, as indicated earlier, the effects are often not immediately apparent, similar to the effects of tobacco, which manifest years and years later. They further reported that glyphosate exposure contributes to cancer, autism, asthma, inflammatory bowel disease, obesity, depression, ADHD, Alzheimer's disease, Parkinson'a disease, ALS, multiple sclerosis, cachexia, infertility, and development malformations.

Scientists generally believe that they can do things better than God can and that God is limited in what he can do for mankind, especially since our population is growing in leaps and bounds and our resources are dwindling just as fast. Maybe if we all lived simply and we all saw ourselves as caretakers, we would be more respectful of the world and its inhabitants and could put into a much clearer perspective whose property we were taking care of. After all, it was here before we got here and it will be here after we are gone. If we could all see this, there would certainly be no more wars because we would all be sharing and trading with each other the resources abundant in our part of the world. It is only due to envy that we wage war. When someone else has what we want and we have the bigger and better weapons or the greater force, we use that force to take it. If God is the owner and we are the caretakers and we, his children, are all brothers and sisters, what would be the need for force?

Aloha!

*

Used in yards, farms and parks throughout the world, Roundup has long been a top-selling weed killer. But now, according to an article in Environmental Health News, written by Crystal Gammon, researchers have found that one of Roundup's inert ingredients can kill human cells, particularly embryonic, placental and umbilical cord cells. Pesticide researchers and activists from the U.S. to Argentina, Japan and Croatia have been calling for public access to, and warnings about, inerts (almost 4,000 solvents, surfactants and other chemicals included in pesticides, approved by the U.S. EPA, yet not specified on warning labels because they are not the "active" ingredient aimed at pest control.)

Glyphosate, Roundup's active ingredient, is the most widely used herbicide in the U.S. About 100 million pounds are applied to U.S. farms and lawns every year. Until now, most health studies have focused on the safety of glyphosate alone, rather than the mixture of ingredients found in Roundup. In a study from the University of Caen, in France, first published earlier this year, scientists found that Roundup's inert ingredients amplified the toxic effect on human cells, even at concentrations much more diluted than those used on farms and lawns. Their focus was on POEA (polyethoxylated tallow amine) an inert detergent in Roundup that they were astonished to discover was far more dangerous than the herbicide itself. The proprietary mixtures available on the market could cause cell damage and even death at the residual levels found on Roundup-treated crops, such as soybeans, alfalfa and corn, or lawns and gardens.

Despite Monsanto's claims that the study is flawed, Giles-Eric Seralini, the molecular biologist that headed the French study, says that standard toxicological methods were used and that competitors can discover what is in formulations like Roundup with routine lab analysis. The purpose of the proprietary protection laws for inerts is solely for the purpose of keeping information from the public. What's worse is that when mixed together at concentrations officially considered "safe," ten of the world's most widely used pesticides can combine to produce a chemical cocktail that is deadlier than any of the chemicals acting alone.

One final note: Monsanto has known since the 1980s that glyphosate causes brain defects and has covered up that piece of information. And in case you know about the chemtrails that are dropping aluminum particles on us, Monsanto has a patent pending for aluminum-resistant seeds. I wouldn't be surprised if Monsanto soon came out with a product called "Soylent Green!"

Everything that I have learned about GMOs I have learned from Jeffery Smith's website: www.instituteforresponsibletechnology.com. Go there. It will blow your mind.

Recently in Hawaii our Senate Agriculture Committee introduced a bill that would require the labeling of all GMO foods. But then, out of the blue, our State Secretary of the Department of Agriculture, former Senator Russell Kokobun, persuaded the Ag Committee to kill the bill because he said that GMOs were safe and posed no danger whatsoever. Gee, why would he do that? Do you think he was motivated by the fact that when he was campaigning as a Senator, he was given $21,000 from Monsanto, DuPont and Pfizer?

All together now – "Pimps, Hookers and Tricks!"

Speaking about genetic modification, I thought you might like to know that in Hawaii we have genetically modified politicians as well. In addition to Kokobun, we have the others that have taken "payoffs" from Monsanto as well:

Our Governor, Neil Abercrombie – he sold out for $1,000.00
Our Speaker of the House, Calvin Say - $1,000.00
Mufi Hanneman, who is running for the US Senate - $1,000.00
House Environmental Protection Committee Member Rep Jerry Chang, $1,000.00
Senate Ag Committee Chairman, Clarence Nishihara – he lost his integrity for $750.00
House Health Committee Chairman, Ryan Yamane - $1,300.00 from Monsanto, Pfizer and AstraZenaca.
House Consumer Protection and Commerce Committee Chairman, Bob Herkes - $1,550.00 from Monsanto and Pfizer.
House Ag Committee Member Cliff Tsuji - $21,500.00 from Monsanto, Syngenta and DuPont.
Former Senator Dwight Takamine, who resigned to work for the Governor - $400.00
Senate Environmental Protection Committee Member Senator,
Mark Nakashima - $500.00
Senate Health Committee Chairman Senator Josh Green - $500.00
Honolulu City Council Chairman, Ernie Martin - $8,000.00

There are actually 65 legislators in all that are genetically modified. But you get the picture as to why GMO labeling bills never make it out of committee.

True environmentalists all!

But, the worst of the worst is Barack Obama. After his victory in 2008, despite his campaign promise to mandatorily label GMOs, he filled key government posts with Monsanto people. Tom Vilsack as head of the Department of Agriculture; Michael Taylor, former vice-president for public policy for Monsanto, as the FDA "food czar; Roger Beachy, former director of the Monsanto Danforth Center, as the director of the National Institute of Food and Agriculture at the USDA; Islam Siddiqui, a former Monsanto lobbyist, as the new Agriculture Trade Representative; Ramona

Romero, the former corporate counsel for DuPont, as the new counsel for the USDA; Rajiv Shah, who held key positions for the Bill and Melinda Gates Foundation, which engages as major funders for GMO research, as the new head of the USAID. Then Hillary Clinton once worked for the Rose law firm, which was counsel to Monsanto, and last but not least, Elena Kagen, nominated by Obama to the US Supreme Court. Had previously argued for Monsanto in the Monanto v. Geertson seed case before the Supreme Court.

Do you really think it was a coincidence that Obama signed the Monsanto Protection Act, AFTER he was elected in 2012? Had he done it before the election there would be someone else in the White House.

Author's Note:

In the recent election (11/12) there was an initiative placed on the California ballot – Proposition 37. Proposition 37 was the initiative to mandatorily label GMO foods.

The "Yes" side was supported by a myriad of organic product companies, Dr Joseph Mercola, the Organic Consumers Association, and the Seed Savers Exchange. They contributed $9 million to the cause.

The "No" side was made up of Monsanto, DuPont, the Grocery Manufacturer's Association, Dow Agro sciences, Bayer, Basf, Syngenta, the Council For Biotechnology Information, the Biotechnology Industry Organization, PepsiCo, Coca Cola, Kraft, Conagra, General Mills, Kellogg, Heinz, Smucker, Rich Products, Unilever, Dean Foods, Abbott Nutrition, Welch's, Tree Top, S&W, and Goya Foods. They raised $47 million.

Before getting into the above a bit deeper, the question you must seriously ask yourself is: If GMOs are as safe as the biotech industry tells us, why did they raise so much money to try to defeat the initiative? And why would these demoniac companies fight so hard to take away our Constitutional right of Freedom of Choice? In order to have a choice, we have to know what is in the food we eat!

Now back to the "NO" guys, many of which control and run organic food companies. How's that for theater of the absurd?

Pepsi controls the IZZE and the NAKED brands; Coca Cola controls the HONEST TEA, ODWALLA, and SIMPLY ORANGE brands; Kraft controls the BACK TO NATURE brand; Conagra controls the LIGHTLIFE and ALEXIA brands; General Mills controls the CASCADIAN FARM ORGANIC, MUIR GLEN, and LARABAR brands; Kellogg controls the KASHI, MORNING STAR FARMS, and GARDENBURGER brands; Heinz is the Ketchup guy; Smucker controls the R.W. KNUDSEN and SANTA CRUZ ORGANIC brands; Unilever controls the BEN & JERRY'S ICE CREAM brand; Dean Foods controls the HORIZON ORGANIC and SILK brands; Rich Products controls the FRENCH MEADOWS BAKERY PRODUCTS brand; Welch's makes the juices; Tree Top controls the TREETOP JUICE brand; Abbott Nutrition controls the SIMILAC brand; S&W controls the S&W brand, and Goya Foods controls the GOYA brand.

Does anyone see the hypocrisy here? These are companies that not only utilize GMOs in their regular products but try to have the best of both worlds by selling organic foods as well.

The bottom line is this: these companies are interested in one thing and one thing only – YOUR MONEY! They could less about your health and well being. Again, you possess only the one thing they want – YOUR MONEY. The best way to avoid giving them your money is to absolutely BOYCOTT their products.

So, here are the rules you must follow to keep your health from deteriorating –

1. You must read the label of every food item you buy.
2. If a food contains soy, corn, or cotton products and the label DOES NOT say organic or non-GMO, DO NOT BUY IT. For example, when you buy an "organic" chocolate bar but the soy lecithin does not say "organic," DO NOT BUY IT.
3. If a product contains canola oil, be it labeled organic or not, DO NOT BUY IT unless you where you can pick a canola.
4. Conventional meat and dairy products come from animals fed GMO grains.
5. If a label says "natural" anywhere, that's a euphemism for GMOs or aspartame or MSG.
6. Magnesium stearate, a common additive in supplements, is derived from GMO corn and soy. DO NOT BUY IT.

7. If you search the *True Food Shoppers Guide*, it will reveal what is in the food you are about to buy.

The rest of what you are about to read will blow your mind. After the election, Proposition 37 lost by 555,000 votes. There was only one thing wrong about that – there were 3.3 million votes that remained uncounted in California. So, how could a win or a loss be determined and who "created" the win?

There are people now that are actively seeking to make sure all votes are counted before a win or a loss can be determined.

Should that answer come to fruition before this book gets published I will come back and include it. Rest assured that Monsanto and their partners in crime are totally responsible for all fabrications. Take back your power and take responsibility by BOYCOTTING these evil entities.

Chapter 4
Process This

Finally, the world cancer experts have declared what people have known for years, that processed meats cause cancer, and anyone seeking to avoid cancer should avoid eating all processed meats for life.

Hundreds of cancer researchers took part in a five-year project spanning more than 7,000 clinical studies and designed to document the links between diet and cancer.

Their conclusion, published in the World Cancer Research Fund's (WCRF) report, 'Food, Nutrition, Physical Activity and the Prevention of Cancer: a Global Perspective' (2007), has rocked the health world with the declaration that: **all people should immediately stop buying and eating processed meat products and that all processed meat should be avoided for life!**

Processed meats, the report explains, are simply too dangerous for human consumption. And why? Because they contain chemical additives that are known to greatly increase the risk of various cancers, including colorectal cancer, breast cancer, prostate cancer, leukemia, brain tumors, pancreatic cancer, and many more. The report also recommends that consumers:

*Avoid all sugary soft drinks for life.
*Exercise at least thirty minutes a day.
*Get lean and fit, without becoming underweight.
*Limit consumption of ALL meats, even fresh meat.
*Breast-feed all infants for their first six months, avoiding infant formula.

Sadly, the WCRF still does not recommend that consumers use nutritional supplements to help protect themselves from cancer, indicating that the group still has a lot to learn about the role of medicinal mushrooms, sea vegetables, microalgae, Chinese herbs, rainforest herbs, super food extracts and organic sulfur crystals in preventing and reversing cancer. At least the group's recommendation that consumers now avoid all processed meat products is a huge step in the right direction. It is the first time any internationally recognized cancer organization has found the courage to make a partial proclamation about the health hazards of the chemicals found in processed meat products. It is almost as big a deal as when the American Medical Association, after years of taking millions of dollars from tobacco companies, finally admitted that smoking causes lung cancer and heart disease. (This was a decade after the scientific evidence was irrefutable, of course, but then again the AMA was making money off Big Tobacco by running ads in JAMA – Journal of the American Medical Association).

There is some doubt in people's minds about the difference between processed meat and non-processed, or "fresh," meat. Here is the difference:

Fresh meat usually has only one ingredient: the meat! Fresh meat is refrigerated and has a very short shelf life, usually just a few days. It is usually packaged in simple wrappers, with no fancy logos or color printing.

Processed meat has many ingredients and is usually packaged for long-term shelf life. These products almost always contain sodium nitrite, the cancer-causing chemical additive that meat companies use as a color fixer to turn their meat products a bright red, "fresh-looking," color. Processed meat products include:

*Bacon
*Sausage
*Pepperoni
*Beef jerky

*Deli slices

*Hot dogs

*Sandwich meat (including those served at restaurants)

*Ham

*Meat "gift' products like Christmas sausages

*Meat used in canned soups

*Meat used in frozen pizza

*Meat used in children's lunch products

*Meat used in ravioli, spaghetti, or Italian pasta products

... and many more meat products.

Unless it says it: "NITRITE FREE" on the front label, you can bet it is made with cancer-causing sodium nitrite!

What Are The Dangerous Chemicals In Processed Meats?

Sodium nitrate is one of the most dangerous chemicals added to processed meats.

Please be aware:

*You MUST read the ingredients list to find the sodium nitrite! Meat product companies do not list this ingredient on the front of the package.

*Even so-called, ORGANIC meat products and NATURAL meat products can still contain sodium nitrate. So read the labels to be sure, and avoid buying any meat products made with sodium nitrate.

*Be especially careful of food for children. Virtually all packaged food products containing meat and marketed to children contains sodium nitrite. Make sure you read the ingredients to protect your child.

Monosodium glutamate (MSG) is a second dangerous chemical found in virtually all processed meat products. MSG is a dangerous excitotoxin linked to neurological disorders such as migraine headaches, Alzheimer's disease, loss of appetite control, obesity and many other serious health conditions. Manufacturers use MSG to add flavor to dead-tasting, processed meat products. (More about MSG in Chapter 10)

Essentially, dead meat products look and taste dead because they are. So meat companies use the following three ingredients to make them look fresh and taste interesting:

Sodium nitrite makes the meat look red and fresh. But, it promotes cancer.

MSG makes the meat taste savory, but it causes neurological disorders.

Processed salt makes the meat taste more interesting, but it causes nutritional problems and high blood pressure.

On top of these three chemical additives, processed meats also contain saturated animal fat that is often contaminated with PCBs, heavy metals, pesticide residues and other dangerous substances.

Processed meats promote cancer. There is simply no question about the scientific validity of that statement, and anyone who disagrees with it is either working for the meat industry or hopelessly behind the times on their nutritional research.

To protect your self from these dangerous processed food products, here are the action steps to take:

1) Check the ingredients of all processed meat products in your refrigerator and pantry.

Throw out any products containing sodium nitrite or monosodium glutamate (MSG).

2) Inform anyone you care about of what you are doing and why you are doing it. Show them the sodium nitrite right on the label of the other products as you throw them out. Let them know that the World Cancer Research Fund now recommends that ALL consumers avoid eating processed meats for life!

3) Boycott all processed meats for life! Never buy processed meats again. That includes shopping at the grocery store, eating at a restaurant, or consuming foods at a social event.

4) Spread the word. Tell others about the dangers of sodium nitrite and MSG. Let people know that processed meats are dangerous for their health.

Something tells me that chemical additives in processed meats are going to emerge as the next big food safety issue to hit mainstream awareness. Just a few years ago, most consumers had never heard of trans fats or the dangers of hydrogenated oils. But once that issue went mainstream, fast food restaurants all over the country announced changes to avoid hydrogenated oils.

More and more consumers are suddenly aware that hotdogs promote cancer, or that bacon consumption is incredibly bad for your health. As awareness of this issue builds, there's going to be increasing political pressure to pass laws that protect the public by strictly limiting or banning the use of sodium nitrite in processed meats.

The meat industry, of course, which seems to have absolutely no respect for human or animal life, will fight this every inch of the way. The people in charge of meat-producing companies exhibit zero concern for the health of the consumers who actually eat their products, and they remain entirely focused on the profits to be had by selling more toxic meat products to gullible consumers.

But, just like Big Tobacco's marketing methods and fraudulent science were finally exposed as wholesale fraud, the processed meat industry is going to have to face scientific facts sooner or later: Sodium nitrite promotes cancer and **eating processed meat products substantially increases your risk of cancer.** There is no denying it or arguing about it, at least not by any sane person. Eating cancer-causing chemicals is blatantly and irrefutably dangerous to your health.

Of course, many low-income, low-education consumers still continue to smoke cigarettes AND eat processed meat products. But the smart consumers, who represent the real future of human civilization are wising up and increasingly opting for healthier foods made WITHOUT dangerous chemicals.

There are people in society today who exhibit a strong desire to commit nutritional suicide. For those people, there will always be beef jerky, hot dogs, frozen pizza, cigarettes and over-hyped "energy" drinks. The future of these people is easy to see: cancer, diabetes, heart disease, chemotherapy, pharmaceuticals, pain, death, and bankruptcy.

Thankfully, there are other people who believe in taking care of their health and in living informed lives with outstanding health. For these people, there are living foods, superfoods, raw cacao, sprouts, rainforest herbs, sunshine, fresh juices and exercise. Their future is also clear: exceptional mental performance, freedom from chronic pain, excellent vitality and longevity, spiritual awareness, abundant living, and much more.

Which group do you want to belong to?

You will make that decision every time you shop for food. When you buy processed meats you will put yourself on a timeline track toward disease, suffering, and medical victimization. But when you avoid meat products and focus on a plant-based diet, you are creating a future filled with abundance and health. It is up to you to decide which of these futures you wish to create.

Regardless of which future you choose, there is no judgment from me. You are free to do what you want with your life and your body. Some people choose to abuse their bodies as chemical playgrounds, living in the moment and dying young. That is their choice. Others choose to extend their lives and honor their bodies, living an extended, purpose-filled life. That's fine too. It's not for me to decide how you live your life. I just want people to live consciously and understand that their decisions create results.

Anyone who decides to eat processed meat products on a repeated basis is simply creating a sad result. That result is cancer. And over enough years that cancer will grow to the point where it shows up on a scan. That's when the doctor says, "You have cancer" and starts prescribing even more toxic chemicals known as chemotherapy agents. This is not a disease with an unknown cause. In fact, cancer is incredibly easy to both prevent AND cure - but only if you understand the fundamentals of nutrition.

For now, just remember:

Processed meats = sodium nitrite = Cancer

If you don't want cancer, don't eat processed meats. Ever!

And if you really want to be healthy, eat a plant-based diet for life.

Another important thing to remember is that young people do not think about getting old. Yet everyone gets old, and many of us develop degenerative diseases. But that's not the point. The point is despite getting old why do we have to feel old? Wouldn't it be nice to get old but not have aches, pains and diseases? That's what a clean and healthy diet provides.

References: Mike Adams' website: www.naturalnews.com
From his article:
"Processed Meat Unsafe for Human Consumption;
Cancer Experts Warn of Dietary Dangers"

Chapter 5

The Great White Hype

Milk is as pure as fresh fallen snow and as familiar as a mother's warm touch. Common sense once led me to believe that if a single food, milk, could sustain a baby as the sole source of nutrients, then it must be "nature's most perfect food". Milk builds strong bones - or so I've been told throughout my life - and since the hardest parts of my body are made mostly of calcium, this liquid must be essential for my strength and stability. Milk is for life, because they tell me I never outgrow my need for milk. All these "facts" were the "truth" until I took the trouble to delve a little deeper. Allow me to share with you what I discovered.

Within the same species - like cow for calf, cat for kitten, mare for foal - mother's milk can be the perfect food for the very young. Not after weaning, for older offspring, and certainly, not the fully-grown. All mammals nourish their developing young with this ready-to-eat liquid, synthesized by specialized sweat glands called the mammary glands. This life-giving fluid contains the nutrients, anti-bodies and hormones that optimize the chances for growth and survival of the infant.

How essential is mother's milk? Human infants deprived of the advantages of human breast milk have:

*Two to four times the risk of sudden infant death syndrome (crib death),
*More than sixty times the risk of pneumonia in the first three months of life,
*Ten times the risk of hospitalization during their first year,
*Reduced intelligence as measured by IQ score,
*Behavioral and speech difficulties,
*An increased chance of suffering from infections, asthma, eczema, Type I diabetes and cancer (lymphoma and leukemia) in early life,
*A greater risk of heart disease, obesity, diabetes, multiple sclerosis, food allergies, ulcerative colitis and Crohn's disease later in life.

No one argues against the fact that human breast milk is nature's most perfect food for human babies. There is also no satisfactory substitute. Therefore, every effort should be made to have every infant breast-fed exclusively for six months, and then, with the addition of healthy solid food choices, breast-fed until the age of two.

The nutritional needs of very young animals are met by the unique qualities of the milk of that particular species. The composition of this infant food has evolved over millions of years to be ideally suited for that animal. Let me explain this in terms of one essential nutrient: protein.

A Human has 1.2 g per 100 ml of protein with a growth rate of 180 days
A Horse has 2.4 g per 100 ml of protein with a growth rate of 60 days
A Cow has 3.3 g per 100 ml of protein with a growth rate of 47 days
A Goat has 4.1 g per 100 ml of protein with a growth rate of 19 days
A Dog has 7.1 g per 100 ml of protein with a growth rate of 8 days
A Cat has 9.5 g per 100 ml of protein with a growth rate of 7 days
A Rat has 11.8 g per 100 ml of protein with a growth rate of 4.5 days

With regard to the grams per 100 ml, in terms of the % of calories, cow's milk has four times more protein than human milk. When you divide the growth rate into the protein you find the cow to be 21% vs. 5% for the human. The growth rate relates to the amount of time it takes to double the birth weight.

It's not rocket science to notice that since the calf doubles its birth weight nearly four times faster than a human infant does, the concentration of protein and calcium are nearly four times greater. This is because rapid growth requires a much higher density of all kinds of nutrients.

The reason that vitamin and mineral supplements are so popular is because most people think of health problems in terms of deficiencies of nutrients. The reality is these diseases are usually due to excess - such as excess dietary fat (obesity), cholesterol (heart disease), and salt (hypertension). Therefore, feeding overly concentrated foods such as cow's milk to people (infants, children, and adults) promotes **diseases of excess.** I'm sure some of you are still thinking that cow's milk corrects calcium deficiency in people, preventing osteoporosis. If you're patient, in a moment I'll show you that this is not true.

Replacing human breast milk with cow's milk was once tried in the mid-1800s, in the United States, for emergency situations such as when a mother died in childbirth. The result was a quick death for most of the infants, because of the high protein content of the cow's milk, which forced fluid losses from the infant's kidneys, resulting in dehydration. Once this problem was recognized, infant formulas were developed, which added sugar to the cow's milk in order to reduce the protein concentration of the cow's milk and make it resemble human milk. Some of you may be old enough to remember drinking infant formula made from Carnation evaporated cow's milk and Karo syrup (sugar). This made for a very unhealthy formula for infants and never should be used.

Consider the purpose of cow's milk: this is an ideal food to grow a calf from its 60-pound birth weight to a 600-pound young cow, ready to wean. This is a "high-octane" fuel. One obvious consequence of people eating "calf food" is rapid weight gain. And dairy products are one of the leading contributors to the epidemic of excess body fat affecting 25% of children and 65% of adults in western populations. Matters are made even worse when cow's milk is converted into even more concentrated products, like cheeses.

Cow's milk products have some important nutritional deficiencies. They are completely devoid of fiber and contain insufficient amounts of vitamins, like C and niacin, and minerals, like iron, to meet the human body's needs.

The dairy industry has spent billions of dollars convincing us that milk is healthy, all the while pumping deadly chemicals into cows and the milk itself.

To think or say that drinking milk is a hype is cause for lynching. Milk, it is said, is "the" source of calcium that helps kids grow up big and strong. Milk is alleged to contain vital nutrients and to help prevent osteoporosis. The US Department of Agriculture, through its food dietary guidelines, says that everyone should get 2-3 servings of dairy every day. Milk is advocated by various government agencies, hordes of physicians, and a $200 million annual advertising budget of the dairy industry. Can we ever forget the mustachioed faces of the countless numbers of celebrities decorating everything from newspaper ads to roadside billboards?

And yes, America has a love affair with milk. So much so that the average person consumes 600 pounds of dairy products every year, including about 420 pounds of fluid milk and cream, 70 pounds of various milk-based fats and oils, 30 pounds of cheese, and 17 pounds of ice cream (obesity epidemic anyone?) In total, the US dairy farmers produce about 15.61 billion pounds of milk and milk products a year. It is "udderly" horrendous, if you'll pardon the pun.

But what if the celebrities we love and trust were lying to us? What if milk doesn't do a body good? What if milk is, instead, a major contributor to breast and prostate cancer, heart disease, asthma, diabetes and more? What if the US government and dairy industry are in bed together to hide the ill effects of dairy consumption? They wouldn't do that, would they?

Well, according to Amy Lanou, PhD., the nutrition director of the Physicians Committee for Responsible Medicine (PCRM), besides the above, "milk has been linked to anemia, allergies, obesity, ovarian cancer, breast-cancer, and juvenile-onset diabetes."

So why, then, is milk regarded as wholesome, especially with the US Department of Agriculture, according to its mission statement, charged with "enhancing the quality of life for the American people by supporting the production of agriculture?"

Created by the pro-business Lincoln administration in 1862, today's USDA has the dual responsibility of assisting dairy farmers while promoting healthy dietary choices for Americans. Would you think that this creates a conflict of interest that puts at risk the objectivity of the government farm policy and the health of the dairy-consuming public? Duh!!

Six of the eleven members assigned to the US Dietary Guidelines Advisory Committee have financial ties to meat, dairy, and egg interests. Prior to the PCRM winning a lawsuit against the USDA, (claiming that it "unfairly promoted the special interests of the meat and dairy industries through its official dietary guidelines and the Food Pyramid"), the USDA refused to disclose such conflicts of interest to the public.

Historically, the USDA's dietary guidelines have consistently reflected the industry's push for greater consumption of both flesh and dairy as evidenced by their concocting the Four Food Groups with milk, meat, fruits and vegetables, and breads and cereals, as the "Big Four" and in that order.

Over the years, these dietary "guidelines" have consistently reflected the industry's push for greater consumption of both meat and dairy, despite the testimony of numerous physicians' groups and watchdog organizations criticizing the Food Pyramid as biased and unhealthy.

The USDA counters this by saying that the guidelines should be "reality-based", arguing that what people should really be eating is moot because it doesn't fit with the American lifestyle. Whaaat? What they are saying is that the USDA doesn't even think it is reasonable to aspire to what constitutes a healthy diet. Now (2011), the psychiatric industry has *invented* a disease called *orthorexia nervosa,* which is Latin for **Healthy Eating Disorder.** It never ends!

May 13, 2002 marked the passage of the farm bill in which dairy farmers and processors received, over 3 1/2 years, an additional $2 billion in subsidies, largely realized through price supports that inflate costs for consumers. Understand that dairy subsidies are a carryover from the Depression era when survival of small dairy farmers was considered essential to maintaining a national food supply. By the way, most of that $2 billion went to larger dairy farms in 12 northeastern states, hanging small farmers out to dry and actually encouraging the demise of family farms.

Another assertion of the suit brought by the PCRM against the USDA is that milk, as a staple in school lunch programs, unfairly discriminates against non-whites who have a high incidence of lactose intolerance. There are about 50 million lactose intolerant adults in the U.S., including 70% of the white population, 95% of blacks, and 80 - 97% of Asian, Native Americans, and Jews of European descent. These 50 million people suffer from a variety of digestive symptoms resulting from milk consumption and other dairy products, including gas, bloating, diarrhea, constipation, and indigestion.

Currently, the USDA requires that every public school in the country serve milk, with the push by some of our elected officials, who benefit greatly by campaign contributions from the dairy industry, to offer financial incentives to schools that installed milk vending machines. To add insult to injury, students cannot get free or subsidized alternatives to milk, like juice or soy milk, or Rice Dream, without a doctor's note. So, for the 70% of the black kids and the 90% of the Asian kids in the public schools, a negative response to lactose intake is practically mandated by the US Government. In essence, these huge dairy subsidies and broad-based promotion of milk by the government's school lunch program is a form of economic racism that isolates minorities and encourages them to ingest something to which they are intolerant or allergic.

Girls in the United States are beginning to menstruate at younger and younger ages. According to the Cancer Prevention Coalition, some girls are now experiencing the effects of puberty as young as three years of age. Fifty years ago, the incidence of breast cancer risk among U.S. women was one in twenty. As of 2001, that percentage has grown to one in eight.

Why is that? Bovine Growth Hormone (BGH)! BGH is a naturally occurring hormone produced by milk cows. Closely resembling the natural growth hormones in human children, the presence of BGH in milk has been shown to significantly elevate hormone levels in people, creating many growth problems. And that's not even accounting for the use of artificial hormones.

Enter Recombinant BGH (rBGH), an unnaturally occurring, genetically modified hormone, produced by Monsanto. As you know, Monsanto has made other fine humanitarian and ecological contributions such as Agent Orange, PCB's, and Roundup laced soy, corn, cotton, canola, sugar beets, and soon with alfalfa, wheat and potatoes.

Through a series of research cover-ups and their network of conflicting interests with government policy makers (and we'll get to that soon), Monsanto, in 1994, managed to get approval for Posilac. This is Monsanto's commercial form of rBGH and increases cow's milk production by 15 to 25%.

According to Monsanto, over a quarter of U.S. milk cows are now in herds supplemented with Posilac. The majority of the country's 1,500 dairy companies mix rBGH with non-rBGH milk during processing to such an extent that an estimated 80 to 90% of the U.S. dairy supply is contaminated.

What Monsanto does not tell consumers is that this supplementation of additional growth hormones is causing secondary sex characteristics to appear earlier in young children, especially girls. Monsanto also does not tell consumers that rBGH injected cows produce extremely high levels of Insulin Growth Factor-1 (IGF-1), a cancer promoter that occurs naturally in the human bloodstream at levels that generally do not result in tumors.

Monsanto and the Fraud and Drug Administration refused the knowledge research directly linking elevated levels of IGF-1 to increased risk of breast and prostate cancer. To make matters worse, Monsanto and the FDA colluded in 1993 and 1994 to block labeling requirements for rBGH milk. Even today Monsanto, the FDA, and the paid-off politicians, block the labeling of genetically modified food. So, the average dairy consumer has no idea that they are increasing their own risk of getting cancer.

Since 1994, every industrialized country in the world, except for the U.S., Canada, Japan, and the 15 nations of the European Union, has banned rBGH milk. Yet, in the face of facts and the majority opinion of the global political and scientific community, Monsanto and the U.S. continued to endorse rBGH milk for general consumption, at the same time trying to figure out why there is an increase in breast cancer deaths as well as the continually declining age of puberty for girls. It's amazing what the Almighty $$$ Sign can accomplish.

It is not rocket science to see that milk is bad for people and that money is more important than concern for the welfare of the people. But what about the effect on the cows that produce that milk? The life expectancy of the average cow under natural conditions is about 25 to 30 years; on the typical factory farm where well over half of the U.S. cows live, they live only 4 to 5 years. Think about how you would feel if your lifespan was decreased by over 80% by people who are only interested in making money.

What happens, because of adding Monsanto's Posilac to the cow's feed, is that it causes them to suffer from mastitis (which is a bacterial infection of the udder), cystic ovaries and uteruses. Aside from the harm to the cows, guess where the pus from the mastitis winds up? Do you now see why drinking milk does **not** do a body good?

By keeping dairy cows constantly pregnant, which is the only way the cow can produce milk, it creates baby calves. Enter the veal industry.

Since the male calves are useless to the farmers and have no economic value, an economic value had to be created. "Hey, let's figure out a way to sell 'em and make money." As the true caring and compassionate farmers that they are, these male calves are taken away from their mothers, immobilized in small wooden crates to keep their flesh tender, and fed fake food so people can "enjoy "their soft flesh after they are slaughtered. In 2001, over 1 million veal calves were slaughtered in the United States. The bottom line is that it boils down to an all-too-familiar story: big business and the U.S. Government joining forces to dupe the American consumer.

The USDA tells us to drink more milk while subsidizing large dairy farms and federally mandating dairy consumption and flesh eating for schoolchildren. The government spends billions to buy unused milk and dairy products, while the industry spends $200 million every year promoting dairy consumption. Meanwhile, the FDA and Monsanto conspire to pollute the already unhealthy dairy supply with a genetically modified hormone banned virtually everywhere else in the world. Ain't the road to profit-at-any- cost, grand?

So, where the American public can answer the absurd industry question, "Got Milk"? with a resounding, mustachioed, "YES," the better question might be to ask whether people have gotten screwed in the process.

In 1990, the Monsanto Company commissioned scientists to inject a bunch of laboratory rats with an early variant of recombinant bovine somatotropin (rBST), a.k.a. rBGH. The 90-day study demonstrated that rBGH was linked to the development of prostate and thyroid cancer in rats. Monsanto, our friend who gave us Agent Orange and spent forty years covering up the effects of PCB's, was about to seek approval for Posilac, that company's form of rBGH. The study linking rBGH to cancer was submitted to the FDA, but somehow in 1994 Posilac was approved. With fingers pointing in both directions, those with opinions argue about who had the bigger part in the cover-up - Monsanto or the Fraud and Drug Administration. The results of this study, in fact, were not made available to the public until 1998, when a group of Canadian scientists obtained the full documentation and completed an independent analysis of the results

Among other instances of neglect, the document showed that the FDA had never even reviewed Monsanto's original studies on which the approval of Posilac had been based.

The FDA's complicity continued; Michael Taylor, a Monsanto lawyer for many years, left in 1976 to become a staff lawyer for the FDA (Taylor was recently appointed by President Obama as the Deputy Commissioner of the FDA). While at the FDA, Taylor also wrote the policy exempting rBGH and other biotech foods from special labeling, considered by most to be a major victory for Monsanto. Ten days after Taylor's policy was finalized, his old law firm, still representing Monsanto, filed suit against two dairy farms that had labeled their milk rBGH free.

As soon as the Government Accounting Office released the report covering all of this, Taylor was removed to work for the USDA, as the Administrator of the Food Safety and Inspection Service, a position he held from 1994 to 1996. After holding positions at both the FDA and the USDA, Taylor went back to working for Monsanto, this time directly as the corporation's Vice President of Public Policy.

Michael Taylor wasn't the only government employee who had this conflict of interest. At the same time Taylor left Monsanto for the FDA,

Dr. Margaret Miller, once Monsanto's top scientist, was also hired by the FDA to review her own scientific research conducted during her tenure at Monsanto. This is so incredible it is worth repeating. A woman who was once Monsanto's top scientist was hired by the FDA to review her own scientific research while she was with Monsanto. So much for "...... and for the people." In her role as FDA scientist, Miller made the official decision to increase the amount of permissible antibiotic residues in milk by a hundred-fold, in part to counter the increase of mastitis in cows due to overuse of artificial growth hormones.

These incestuous relationships between industry and the U.S. Government are the norm rather than the exception. Decisions at the FDA are made primarily by advisory boards comprised of scientists and executives from the dairy and meat industries, with a few university academics thrown in for good measure.

In July of 2010, the "Terminator," California's Governor Arnold Schwarzenegger, signed the bill that would essentially prohibit, starting in 2015, any egg from being sold in the state that comes from caged hens. The bill became law twenty months after a majority of California voters approved Proposition 2, making it clear that concern for the living conditions of livestock is no longer the province of animal rights activists alone.

Recognizing how widespread concern about the humane treatment of farm animals has become, the California Milk Advisory Board has recently ramped its ten-year "Happy Cow" advertising campaign with a new series of ads proclaiming that, "Great milk comes from Happy Cows. Happy Cows come from California." These ads are now being shown across the nation. Unfortunately, there are a few problems with the ads. For one, they weren't filmed in California at all. They were filmed in Auckland, New Zealand, and that's just the tip of the iceberg.

Current Milk Board ads claim that 99% of the state's dairy farms are family owned. But, in order to arrive at this figure, they count as "dairy farms," rural households with one or two cows. Meanwhile, there are corporate-owned dairies in the San Joaquin Valley which have 15,000 or 20,000 cows. It is these far larger enterprises that produce the vast majority of California's milk.

My concern, let me emphasize, is not with the small-scale farms. I have no problem with the many hard-working families who treat their cows well, take care of the land and try to bring a healthy product to market. My problem is with the much larger agribusiness enterprises, the factory farms to whom the animals in their care are nothing but sources of revenue.

Thanks to the practices they employ, the amount of milk produced yearly by the average California cow is nearly 3000 pounds more than the national average. This increased production may seem like a good thing, but is achieved at great cost to the animals. The cows are routinely confined in extremely unnatural conditions, injected with hormones, fed antibiotics, and generally treated with all the compassion of four-legged milk pumps. Roughly one-third of California's cows suffer from painful udder infections, and more than half suffer from other infections and illnesses.

Although genetically engineered bovine growth hormone is banned in many countries including Canada, Australia, New Zealand, and much of the European Union, it is widely used in California's largest dairy operations to increase milk production. Unfortunately, it also increases udder infections and lameness in the cows, markedly raises the amount of pus found in milk, and may increase the risk of cancer in consumers.

The natural lifespan of a dairy cow is about twenty-five years, but one-fourth of California's dairy cows are slaughtered each year (typically at four or five years old), because they've become crippled from painful infections or calcium depletion, or simply because they can no longer produce the unnaturally high amounts of milk required of them. The Milk Board ads present the California dairy industry as a bucolic enterprise that operates in lush, grassy pastures. Some of the ads employ the slogan, "So much grass, so little time." Here, the cows are typically kept in overcrowded dirt feedlots. Some never see a blade of grass in their entire lives.

The ads show calves in meadows talking happily to their mothers. But the calves born to California dairy cows typically spend only twenty-four hours with their mothers, and some do not even get that much.

The ads propagate the image that California dairy cows live in natural conditions and the practices of the dairy industry are in harmony with the environment. But the amount of excrement (doo doo) produced each year by the dairy cows in the fifty-square mile area of California's Chino

Basin would make a pile of doo doo equaling the dimensions of a football field and as tall as the Empire State building. When it rains heavily, dairy manure in the Chino Basin is washed straight into the Santa Ana River and some makes its way into the aquifer that supplies half of Orange County's drinking water.

The large-scale factory dairies in California's Central Valley produce more excrement then the entire human population of Texas. About twenty-million Californians (65% of the state's population) rely on drinking water that is threatened by contamination from nitrates and other poisons stemming from the dairy manure. Nitrates have been linked to cancer and birth defects.

The Milk Board defends the ads by saying they are entertaining, and "are not intended to be taken seriously." But the Milk Board is not in the entertainment business. It has not spent hundreds of millions of dollars on this ad campaign to amuse the public, but to increase the sales of California dairy products. Besides, does misleading the public become legitimate just because it is done in an entertaining way?

The Milk Board knows that showing calves being taken away from their bellowing mothers and being confined in tiny veal crates will not sell their product. Neither will showing emaciated, lame animals, who have collapsed from a lifetime of hardship and over-milking, being taken to slaughterhouses and having their throats slit. But this is the reality for animals in the large-scale factory farms that produced most of the state's milk. Covering up his misery with fantasy ads of happy cows who are actually in New Zealand is not amusing. It is perpetrating a sham on the public.

This is why I have joined with People for the Ethical Treatment of Animals (PETA) in a lawsuit that challenges the Milk Board's ads as unlawfully deceptive. Thus far, the Milk Board has prevailed in court, even though it is obvious that the ads lied to the public. Why? Because the California Milk Advisory Board is the marketing arm of the California Department of Agriculture, a government agency. And in California, in a truly Orwellian twist, Government agencies are exempt from laws prohibiting false advertising.

Should we hold our advertisers, even if they are government agencies, accountable to reality? Should we require that what they tell us has some resemblance to the truth?

Recently, PETA has erected billboards throughout the state that read, "California Cheese Comes From Miserable Cows". PETA, of course, is an animal rights group, but this issue is increasingly being recognized as one that concerns not only vegetarians or vegans or animal advocates. Consumers who want the animal products they buy to be from humanely raised animals can be found in every segment of the society.

Consideration for the plight of animals is a central part of the American character. It is an essential part of who we are as a people. The "Happy Cow" ads are an insult to the legitimate humanitarian concerns of millions of people. As consumers, do we want to reward this sort of behavior with our hard-earned dollars?

Abraham Lincoln was speaking not only for vegetarians or vegans or animal rights advocates when he said, "I care not much for a man's religion whose dog or cat are not the better for it."

A word of good advice to adhere to: If a product originally had a face or a mother or if man made it and you can't pronounce it, don't eat it!

We live in a world governed by greed, dishonesty and lack of compassion. To survive, we must rely on our innate intelligence and do what our bodies tell us. We must shake ourselves free from the pharmaceutical-medical-insurance cartel and put the control of our health back into our hands. We, in order to achieve good health and a good quality of life, must transcend the endless messages we are bombarded with through the various media outlets and be sensible. To get on the road to recovery, we must eliminate those causes from touching our lips. Flesh foods, found in anything that walks, runs, flies, crawls or swims, and dairy products, are loaded with artery clogging saturated fat. Processed foods, refined grains (white, in this case, is not right), sugary foods like sodas, cookies, cakes, doughnuts, and eggs, have to go. The yolks of the eggs are high in cholesterol and the whites, because of their hardening affect, are used as a base in aircraft paint because they can withstand the effects of extreme weather conditions. If you don't believe me and you still eat eggs, the next time you do so, don't wash your dish for a day or two and see what happens. And after you have to scrape it off your plate with a chisel or a screwdriver you might want to think about whether or not you want to continue putting this into your body.

Take time to prepare your own meals, slow down, try to relax, and engage in a meditation practice. There are so many avenues of education available to you. Life is too short to not make the most of it and only you can make you truly well. You are your own best investment. Let today be the day you take your first step in the marathon of life.

References: Reprinted with permission By Dr. John McDougall and John Robbins
From part of Dr. McDougall's article,
"Dairy Products and 10 False Promises"
From John Robbins article: "Happy Cows? Hardly!"

The rest is from my gathering of information during my 30 + years on the radio.

P.S. The dairy industry has recently petitioned the FDA to add artificial sweeteners such as aspartame and Splenda to all milk sold in stores without requiring any labeling of such. So, instead of just getting a white liquid devoid of any nutrition due to pasteurization, homogenization, GMO growth hormones added, antibiotics, and pus, now you can get neurological disorders as well. Some people never learn!

Chapter 6

Dump "Humpty"

Eggs are the richest unprocessed food commonly consumed. Rational thinking people might partake of this delicacy on a special occasion, such as after the annual Easter egg hunt.

Any reasonable behavior is undermined by the American Egg Board whose mission it is to make every day Easter for everybody. The board has a $14 million annual budget to accomplish this job. According to their website (www.enc-online.org), "The American Egg Board's mission is to allow egg producers to fund and carry out proactive programs to increase markets for eggs, egg products and spend money for fowl products through promotion, research and education."

As the egg industry's promotion arm, the American Egg Board's foremost challenge is to convince the American public that the egg is still "one of nature's most perfect foods." Their efforts are working: US egg production during 2003 was 73.93 billion table eggs. This means, on average, 235 eggs a year for every single man, woman and child in the country.

The purpose of a hen's egg is to provide all the materials necessary to develop the one cell - created by the joining of a cock's sperm, with the hen's ova - into a complete chick with feathers, beak, legs, and tail. This miraculous growth and development is supported by a 1-1/2 ounce package of ingredients - a hen's egg - jam-packed with proteins, fats, cholesterol, vitamins and minerals. As a result, the hen's egg has been called, "one of nature's most nutritious creations."

Indeed, an egg is the richest of all foods, and far too much of a "good thing" for people. The components of a cooked egg, even a hard-boiled egg, are absorbed through our intestines. As a result, this highly concentrated food provides too much cholesterol, fat and protein for our body to process safely. The penalties are *diseases of over nutrition* - heart disease, obesity, and type-2 diabetes to name only a few consequences from malnutrition due to the SAD (Standard American Diet).

Eggs are promoted as the ideal source of protein for people and often referred to as a "perfect protein." Eggs are indeed high in protein, but the kinds of proteins in hen's eggs are not ideal for people. In one study, volunteer subjects were fed different foods to determine the ability of humans to utilize various protein mixtures. Investigators found that our bodies can utilize the proteins in a mixture of eggs and potatoes 36% more efficiently than those from eggs alone.

If the protein make-up of eggs were ideal, then you couldn't improve upon it by adding potatoes, could you? Vegetable sources provide for all the protein needs of people and are much safer and more ideal than from hen's eggs.

A whole egg is 32% protein and the white of the egg is essentially 100% protein. Infants, growing children and adults need, at most, 5% of their calories from protein. Therefore, eggs and egg products are six to twenty times more concentrated in protein than we need. Excess protein places burdens on your body, especially on organs of metabolism, the liver and kidneys. Animal proteins, and particularly those from egg whites, are high in troublesome, sulfur-containing amino acids, such as methionine.

Here are six examples of how excess sulfur-containing amino acids in your diet can adversely affect your health:

1) Amino acids, as the name implies, are acids; the sulfur-containing amino acids are the strongest acids of all, because they break down into

powerful **sulfuric** acid. Excess dietary acid is a primary cause of bone loss leading to osteoporosis and kidney stone formation.

2) The sulfur-containing amino acid methionine is metabolized into *homocysteine.* This substance is a risk factor associated with heart attacks, strokes, peripheral vascular disease, venous thrombosis, dementia, Alzheimer's disease, and depression.

3) Sulfur feeds cancerous tumors. (Note: the sulfur referred to in this article is not to be confused with organic sulfur crystals, which will be further explained in another chapter). Cancerous cell metabolism is dependent upon methionine being present in the diet, whereas normal cells can grow on a methionine-free diet (feeding off other sulfur-containing amino acids).

4) Sulfur from sulfur-containing amino acids is known to be toxic to the tissues of the intestine, and have deleterious effects on the human colon, even at low levels - possibly causing ulcerative colitis.

5) Restriction of methionine in the diet has been shown to prolong the life of experimental animals.

6) Halitosis, body odor, and noxious flatus - akin to the smell of rotten eggs - are direct results of the sulfur-containing amino acids that we eat. The foul odors of sulfur gases should be a clear message that something is terribly wrong and deserves our immediate attention.

A significant amount of the $14 million collected each year by the American Egg Board is allocated for research projects, examining the effects of dietary cholesterol on serum cholesterol levels in order to prove that eating eggs will not raise your risk of dying of heart disease. This is quite an endeavor when you consider that eggs are the most concentrated source of cholesterol in the human diet - eight times more cholesterol than beef. Traditionally, in scientific studies on humans, eggs have been used as the source to demonstrate the adverse effects of cholesterol on our health and our heart arteries.

Dozens of papers published in scientific journals and funded by "The Egg Nutrition Center" and/or the "American Egg Board," downplay the hazards of eating eggs. So how do they demonstrate that eating loads these cholesterol-filled delicacies has little effect on blood cholester

The trick is to saturate the subjects with cholesterol from other sources, like beef, chicken, and/or fish and then add eggs to the person's diet. Once a person has consumed 400 to 800 mg of cholesterol in the day, adding more (like an egg) causes little rise because the bowel cannot absorb much more cholesterol. Poor-quality studies, often funded by the egg industry, add to the false information they use to vindicate their products. The actual impact of egg feeding is seen when people who eat little cholesterol are fed eggs. When seventeen lacto-vegetarian college students, consuming 97 mg of cholesterol daily, were fed one extra-large egg daily for three weeks their "bad" LDL-cholesterol increased by 12%.

The real-life effects of eggs were recently investigated in a large population of nearly 6000 vegetarians and 5000 non-vegetarians over a period of thirteen years. Within this group of nearly 11,000 people, those eating eggs more than six times a week had a 2.47 times greater risk of dying of heart disease than those eating less than one egg a week.

A fifty-year study of nearly 2000 middle-aged men, the Western Electric Study, found that dietary reduction and cholesterol intake of 430 mg/dl (same as 2 eggs) was associated with a 43% reduction in long-term risk of coronary heart disease, a 25% reduction of risk of death from all causes, and three years longer life expectancy. In addition to heart disease, higher cholesterol intake is also associated with more risk of strokes, blood clots, high blood pressure and cancers of the breast, prostate, colon, lung, and brain. Cholesterol is the most damaging to our arteries when it is present in an oxidized form, as free radicals. Eggs and egg-derived products are the main source of oxidized cholesterol in our diet.

Untainted research from high-quality studies shows that adding one egg to the daily diet of the average "healthy" person, already eating 200 mg of cholesterol from other sources, will increase their serum cholesterol by about 4%, which translates into an 8% increase in their risk of heart disease. Two eggs daily will mean a 6% increase in cholesterol and 12% more hea~~ ~~ over the next 5 to 10 years. For young men, indulgence ~~aster Bunny treats" daily, means a 30% higher risk of ~~se over their lifetime.

~~th too much protein, cholesterol, calories, fat, bacteria, ~~hemical contamination, to be consumed with any frequency, with any expectation of health. Egg protein is a common source of allergy in infants, children and adults, producing problems from hives to asthma. Eggs are high in fat, which promotes obesity and type-2 diabetes. Fats and cholesterol in eggs promote the formation of cholesterol gallstones and gallbladder attacks.

Egg-borne infections caused by salmonella bacteria can give rise to cramps, diarrhea, nausea, vomiting, chills, fever and/or headache and food poisoning - called salmonellosis. Eggs are a main contributor to human exposure to dioxin and other environmental chemicals that are known to cause birth defects, neurological damage, and cancer. Many nutritional qualities of eggs are similar to the nutritional qualities of cow's milk, cheese, chicken, beef, and fish - foods known to cause major health problems when consumed in the typical amounts of people living in western societies.

Twenty-five years ago, based on the concerns of the American Heart Association, the Federal Trade Commission carried out legal action, upheld by the US Supreme Court, to compel the egg industry to desist from false and misleading advertising, claiming that eggs had no harmful effects on health. These days, with a $12 million annual budget for product promotion, matters are even worse than before, with the egg industry now making unrestrained claims like:

"There is no need to avoid eggs on a heart-healthy diet"

"Even cholesterol-lowering diets allow moderate amounts of whole eggs"

"An egg a day may keep heart disease away"

"Eat your eggs, they're good for you"

Unfortunately, we live in a " lawless wild west" when it comes to consumer protection from the big food businesses. Therefore, only you can defend yourself and your family from such profit- driven bogus claims and the harms that come with them.

References: www.drmcdougall@dr.mcdougall.com
From Dr. McDougall's article,
"Eggs Are For Easter"

One final note for egg eaters:

After you cook and eat eggs, do not wash your plate or frying pan for a day. Then when you find that you need to use a chisel to scrape the eggs off the plate and frying pan, you will realize that what happened to your plate and pan is what happens to your arteries. And as your consumption continues and your arteries become more constricted due to the buildup, you will have to admit that you, and only you, are responsible for the heart attack that could one day hit you.

Chapter 7

Beat Your Meat. Habit

Human beings have been consuming meat as part of their diet for most of their existence and will likely continue this behavior until the last living animal is gone from the earth.

Public awareness, however, of meat-associated health hazards, such as heart attacks, colon cancer, and fatal E. coli bacterial infections, has caused great concern and shifts in many people's eating habits. The number of vegetarians has been growing worldwide, especially among better-educated and younger people. An astonishing contradiction to this trend was a very popular weight loss diet - the Atkins Diet - which was almost entirely meat. Obviously, there was much disagreement and confusion. And, by the way, Dr. Atkins dropped dead of a heart attack on the sidewalk in New York City.

There is no more important question to be answered for mankind than, "What is the proper diet for human beings?" What is the diet that allows us to look, feel, and function at our best, not just to survive or lose weight? Is it vegetarian? Does it contain flesh? How much flesh? There must be a correct answer. Just like there was one diet best for horses, one for cats, one for dogs and one for each kind of bird - there must be one best for people.

Why have we not discovered this diet? It is certainly not because of lack of interest. Russell Henry Chittenden, the father of American biochemistry and professor of physiological chemistry at Yale Medical School, wrote, a century ago (1904), "We hear on all sides widely divergent views regarding the needs of the body, as to the extent and character of food requirements, contradictory statements as to the relative merits of animal and vegetable foods. Indeed, there is a great lack of agreement regarding many of the fundamental questions that constantly arise in any consideration of the nutrition of the human body."

You would think that after so many years of investigation using the latest scientific methods and employing modern technology that this matter of such grave importance would have been settled beyond a doubt. Today's coexistence of enthusiastic advocates of "all meat" and "no meat" diets, and everything in between, prove this matter is far from settled.

Dr. John McDougall states: "Regardless of how much other doctors may argue the merits of their opinions on the best diet (supported, of course, by the latest "facts"), they do not have the same glowing outcomes with their patients - I have seen the consequences. For me, as a practicing doctor, the bottom line is *patient results.* Fortunately, there is an overwhelming amount of undeniable scientific data and observations clearly supporting my conclusions."

"Many scientists use the diet of our ancestors as the justification for what we should eat today. This may be a useful approach, but which ancestors are we to follow? Differences of opinion arise because throughout human history people have consumed a wide variety of foods. The early ancestors of modern humans, from at least 4 million years ago, followed diets almost exclusively of plant-foods. Beginning at least 250,000 years ago, many of the hunter-gatherer societies consumed meat as a large part of their diet. However, more recently, over the past 12,000 years of agricultural development, people's diets have been mostly based upon starches, like rice in Asia, corn in North America, potatoes in western parts of South America, wheat in Europe and Northern Africa. In terms of the time line of evolution, 12,000 years, and even 250,000 years, is only a brief moment."

The Bible story of Adam and Eve's eviction from the Garden of Eden is closely analogous to the actual shift from early plant-eating humans to hunter-gatherer's. While in the Garden, God said," I give you every seed-bearing plant on the face of the whole earth and every tree that has fruit with seed in it. They will be your meat". Upon expulsion, humans were instructed by God, "By the sweat of your brow you will earn your food".

For the most part, hunter-gatherers, like the exiles from the Garden, had a subsistence standard of living, eating foods that extended from one extreme to the other in their proportions of plants vs. animal foods: from the raw flesh and the fat of marine mammals - the Arctic Eskimos - to diets composed largely of wild plants of the western diet of the Australian Aborigines. Hunter-gatherers took advantage of any dependable sources of food from their wild local environments. Because of the ease and dependability (compared to obtaining animals) the gathering of fruits and vegetables was a primary source of food for most hunter-gatherer societies. The emphasis on hunting increases in higher latitudes because of plant scarcity.

Undoubtedly, all of these diets were adequate to support growth and life to an age of successful reproduction. To bear and raise offspring you only need to live for twenty to thirty years, and fortuitously, the average life expectancy for these people was just that. The few populations of hunter-gatherers surviving into the 21st Century are confined to the most remote regions of our planet - like the Arctic and the jungles of South America and Africa - some of the most challenging places to survive. Their life expectancy is also limited to twenty-five to thirty years and infant mortality is 40% to 50%. Hunter-gatherer societies did survive, but considering their arduous struggle and short life span, they cannot be ranked among successful societies.

So why has meat been an important part of the diet for so many of these hunter-gatherer societies? Throughout human history, especially before the development of agriculture-based living, acquiring food for survival was a full-time job. Food scarcity, even starvation, plagued most of these people, at least some of the time. Meat represented a gold mine of concentrated calories and nutrients whenever it was obtained. For those societies who found a plentiful supply, survival on a meat-based diet simply attests to the resilience and adaptability of the human frame.

However, the fact that many hunter-gatherer societies obtain most of their calories from the fat of meat, does not mean meat is the ideal diet for modern people. Almost every scientist readily admits that the composition of wild game available to our ancestors was far different from the grain-fed, domesticated high-fat meat that people eat these days. Furthermore, even if humans have been eating meat for centuries, this has not been with the kind of ease which wealthy westerners acquire it today. Without refrigeration and other means of preserving meat in a near fresh state, consumption is limited to within a few days of the kill -until the meat spoiled. With the advent of fire, people learn to preserve meat by smoking it.

During difficult times, meat provided more benefits than harms. But in a society where food is plentiful and life is physically easy, meat can become a serious health hazard. A traditional Arctic Eskimo, living in a subfreezing climate, could expend 6000 calories and more a day just to keep warm and hunt for food. The high-fat animal food sources - fish, walrus, whale, and seal - from his local environment were the most practical means of meeting the demands of those rigorous surroundings. Modern Eskimos, living in heated houses and driving around in their climate-controlled SUVs, still consuming a high-meat diet, have become some of the fattest and sickest people on earth. Of course, they now use a "green lure" (a $10 bill) to catch their fish (sandwich).

Evolution in the animal kingdom dates back hundreds of millions of years and the evolution of humans began over four million years ago. The ancestors of modern humans were believed to live primarily on plant foods, eating wild fruits, leaves, roots, and other high quality plant parts with a few animal foods in their daily diet.

These pre-humans ate like our nearest primate relatives, the apes of today. Now, biologists at Wayne State University School of Medicine in Detroit, Michigan, provide new genetic evidence that lineages of chimpanzees and humans diverged so recently that chimps should be reclassified as members of our genus, *Homo*, along with Neanderthals, and all other human-like fossil species. "We humans appear as only slightly remodeled chimpanzee-like apes," says the study.

Most apes living today eat essentially as vegetarians - consuming a diet comprised of fruits, leaves, flowers, and bark, with sporadic consumption of very small amounts of insect materials, like termites, and less commonly, small animals. These meat-eating activities may be purely social in nature and unrelated to any real nutritional needs.

Behavior can be changed overnight, but our anatomy and physiology only evolve from selective pressures of the environment over millions of years. Food is the strongest contact with our environment. Therefore, the present state of the human body accurately reflects how our kind has eaten during most of our human and pre-human existence. These indisputable anatomical and physiological characteristics clearly identify the best diet for people today.

"Heshie, eat your beef, you have to get your protein." Worried about her growing child, my mother said this to me at almost every dinnertime. "But ma, it's hard to chew." So, I did the best I could but eventually swallowed big chunks. After a while, I simply gave the pieces of beef to my dog Tippy, who was sitting under the table.

Our teeth evolved for processing starches, fruits, and vegetables, not tearing and chewing flesh. Our oft-cited "canine" teeth are not at all comparable to the sharp teeth of true carnivores. Ask a dentist to show you the "canine" teeth in your mouth that resemble a cat's or dog's "canine "teeth" and you'll grow old waiting to see those sharply pointed ones.

If you have any doubt of the truth of this, then go look in the mirror right now. Maybe you've learned to call your four corner front teeth, "canine teeth," but in no way do they resemble the sharp, jagged blades of the true carnivore. Your corner teeth are short, blunted, and flat on top, or slightly rounded at most. Not only that, but they never function in the manner of true canine teeth. Have you ever seen somebody purposefully favoring those teeth while tearing off a piece of steak or chewing it? Me neither. The lower jaw of the meat-eating animal has very little side-to-side motion. It is fixed to open and close, which adds strength and stability to its powerful bite. Like other plant-eating animals, our jaw can move forward and backwards, side-to-side, as well as open and closed, for biting off pieces of plant matter, and then grinding them into smaller pieces with our flat molars.

In a failed attempt to chew and swallow pieces of food, usually meat, approximately 4000 people die each year in the U.S. They choke on inadequately chewed chunks of flesh that become stuck in their throats.

The Heimlich maneuver was specifically designed to save the lives of people dying from these stuck pieces of flesh and bones.

From our lips to our butts, our digestive system has evolved to efficiently process plant foods. Digesting begins in the mouth with a salivary enzyme called ptyalin, whose sole purpose is to help digest the complex carbohydrates found in plant foods, into simple sugars. There are no carbohydrates in meats of any kind. So, a true carnivore has no need for this enzyme as their salivary glands do not synthesize ptyalin.

The stomach juices of a meat-eating animal are very concentrated in acid. The purpose of this acid is to efficiently break down the muscle and bone materials swallowed in large quantities into the stomachs of meat-eaters. Digestion of starches, vegetables and fruits are accomplished efficiently with the much lower concentration of stomach acid found in the stomachs of humans and other plant-eaters.

The human intestine is long and coiled, much like that of apes, cows, and horses. This configuration makes digestion slow, allowing time to break down and absorb the nutrients from plant food sources. The intestine of a carnivore, like a cat, is short, straight, and tubular. This allows for very rapid digestion of flesh and excretion of the remnants quickly before they putrefy and rot. There are also marked sacculations, which are many sac-like enlargements that bulge out along the large intestine, like those found in all apes, which strongly supports the view that we are primarily plant-eating animals. Overall, the intestines of meat-eaters are noticeably simpler than ours.

Cholesterol is only found in animal foods - no plant contains cholesterol. The liver and biliary system of a meat-eating animal has an unlimited capacity to process and excrete cholesterol from his body: it goes out in the bile, passing through the bile ducts and gallbladder, into the intestine, and finally, out with the stool. For example, you can feed a dog or cat pure egg yolks all day long and they will easily get rid of all of it and never suffer from a backup of cholesterol. Humans, like other plant-eating animals, have livers with very limited capacities for cholesterol removal: they can remove only a little more than they make for themselves for their own bodies. As a result, most people have great difficulty eliminating the extra cholesterol they take in from eating animal products. The apparent "inefficiency" is because humans have evolved on a diet of mostly plant foods (containing no cholesterol). Therefore, they never required a highly efficient cholesterol-biliary system. The resulting cholesterol buildup, when people eat meat, causes deposits in the arteries (atherosclerosis), in the skin under the eyes, (xanthelasma), and in the tendons. Bile, supersaturated with cholesterol, forms gallstones (over 90% of gallstones are made of cholesterol). About half of all middle-aged women who live on the western diet have cholesterol gallstones.

To believe we require the body parts of other animals in our diet for good health pre-supposes the human body evolved over millions of years on a diet predominantly of meat and deficient in plants. This is not what is seen when the nutritional requirements of people are examined.

When plants have been, for eons, a plentiful and reliable part of the diet, an animal can become dependent upon specific nutrients found in these foods. For example, ascorbic acid, found preformed and ready to use in plant foods, is called vitamin C in the diet of people. Insufficient amounts of this vitamin causes scurvy. Vitamins are essential micronutrients that cannot be synthesized by the body; and therefore, must be in the food. Because ascorbic acid has not been readily available to them, meat- eating animals have retained the ability to synthesize ascorbic acid from basic raw materials found in their meat diet. Therefore, it is not a vitamin for them. In other words it is not "vital" or essential to be preformed in their food supply.

Because humans have lived throughout most of their evolution on diets with very little animal matter, they have had to develop or retain the ability to synthesize some substances they need that are abundantly found in meat. For example, humans and other plant-eating animals, have the ability to make vitamin A from a precursor found in large quantities in plants, called beta-carotene. Carnivores cannot utilize beta-carotene as a precursor of vitamin A. They have no need to; throughout their evolution they have always had a plentiful supply of preformed vitamin A (Retinol) found in the meat. Carnivores have also lost the ability to synthesize Niacin, which is plentiful in meat. Remember, efficiency is necessary for survival of the species and it is inefficient to keep manufacturing processes in the body that are useless.

For most enlightened people in modern western nations, the idea of chasing down and killing an animal is revolting, and the thought of consuming that freshly killed flesh is repulsive. To eat decaying flesh, as a vulture does, would be next to impossible. Even when meat is cooked, most people are disgusted by the thought of eating a slice of horse, kangaroo, rat, or cat. Cows, chickens and pigs are acceptable to most westerners only because we have eaten them all our lives. Yet even then, to make meat palatable, its true nature must be covered up with a strong flavored sauce made with salt, sugar, and/or spices - like sweet and sour, marinara, barbecue, or steak sauce. Few people enjoy boiled beef or chicken.

People do not have a negative reaction to unfamiliar fruits and vegetables. I could ask you to try an unfamiliar "star fruit" from Hawaii for the first time and you would eat and enjoy it without hesitation. Why? Because your natural instincts are to eat fruits and vegetables.

So, many human characteristics clearly indicate we have evolved to be primarily plant-eaters. Our hands are made for gathering plants, not ripping flesh. We cool ourselves by sweating, like most other plant-eating animals. Carnivores cool their bodies by panting. We drink our beverages by sipping, not lapping like a dog or cat. The exhaustive factual comparisons of our bodily traits with that of other animals prove that we have evolved over eons in an environment of plant-based foods. The only real contradiction is our behavior. The results of our aberrant behavior can be catastrophic. Let me give you an example of that harm regarding macho men.

Men traditionally have been the hunters who carry back the slain animals to feed the village. You know, "They bring home the bacon!" Scientific research confirms that meat is viewed as a superior masculine food. The acts of killing, butchering and eating animals are associated with power, aggression, virility, strength, and passion - all attributes desired by most men. And, eating meat has long been associated with aggressive behaviors and violent personalities. Men say they need more, and they do eat more meat (especially more red meat), then women. However, based on male anatomy real men should be vegetarians.

Human males have seminal vesicles. No other meat-eating animal has these important collecting-pouches as part of their reproductive anatomy. The seminal vesicles are paired sacculated pouches connected to the prostate, located at the base of the bladder. They collect fluids made by the prostate that nourish and transports the sperm. Ejaculation occurs when the seminal vesicles and prostate empty into the urethra of the penis. In many ways, masturbation is the ultimate act of male performance.

Eating meat diminishes sexual performance and masculinity. The male hormone, testosterone, that determines sexual development and interest has been found to be 13% higher in vegans. Meat-eaters are likely to become impotent because of damage caused to the artery system that supplies their penises with the blood that causes an erection. Erectile dysfunction is more often seen in men with elevated cholesterol levels and high levels of LDL "bad cholesterol" - both conditions related to habitual meat-eating.

The greatest threat to a man's virility is from the high levels of environmental chemicals concentrated in modern meats of all kinds. These chemicals interfere with the actions of testosterone. Decreased ejaculate volume, low sperm count, shortened sperm life, poor sperm motility, genetic damage, and infertility result from eating meat with estrogen-like environmental chemicals. These chemicals in the meat, eaten by his mother, influence a smaller penis and testicles, as well as deformity of the penis and undescended testicles. Estimates are that 89% to 99% of the chemical intake into our body is from our food, and most of this is from foods high on the food chain - meat, poultry, fish, and dairy products.

The enlightened diet for humans today is centered around starchy plant foods with the addition of fruits and vegetables. **If your diet deviates too far from that which has evolved over eons of time then you will likely suffer serious consequences. These are the chronic diseases affecting people living on the western diet.**

References: drmcdougall@drmcdougall.com
From Dr. McDougall's article,
"Meat in the Human Diet"

Remember in the GMO chapter I told you about a "babooz" named Russell Kokobun? But wait, there's more...

On the west side of Honolulu there is a closed-down, dilapidated slaughterhouse that has lost money since its inception. Recently, there was a hearing at our capitol where our House Finance Committee heard a bill to resurrect that slaughterhouse. Twenty or so people, including myself, went to testify against the bill. There were over 300 written testimonies opposing the bill as well. Every time an opposing testimony was given, the person was met with, "speed it up," or "there's a three minute limit," or "sum it up now."

Enter Russell Kokobun and some jerk from the Cattlemen's Association. They both ranted about how essential it was to reopen the slaughterhouse and have the State of Hawaii own, operate and refurbish it to the tune of $1.6 million. The Committee hung onto their every word, let them talk as long as they liked, and basically ignored the 320 plus opposing testimonies. The worst part, well actually two worst parts, is that the slaughterhouse would be the ONLY state-owned and run slaughterhouse in the entire United States. The next worst part is that our State Secretary of Agriculture, Kokobun, can be bought by anyone. When I heard that this concept was pushed so heavily by the Cattlemen's Association, I asked the Committee why the Cattlemen's Association didn't undertake the project themselves instead of pushing it upon the State? It was as if I were not even in the room.

Once again, all together now - "Pimps, Hookers and Tricks!"

Chapter 8

Fowl Ball

C hicken and turkey are called "white meats" as in "clean white meat", and are considered to be "health foods". The truth is that fowl are filthy with a multitude of disease-causing ingredients. The horrible threat of a bird flu pandemic may cause health-conscious people to examine more closely the facts behind this traditional meal centerpiece. We may see something similar to the way mad cow disease, with all the emotions it aroused, caused people to rethink beef. To date, only a handful of people have died from either of these animal-borne infections, yet the fear of these two diseases could save millions of lives as people refrain from eating the more ordinary, but very lethal, parts of an animal's tissues.

The tissues of all fowl contain artery-clogging fat and cholesterol, and bone-destroying protein and acid. They are completely devoid of energy-giving carbohydrate and bowel-moving fiber. Like "sauce on the goose" they are contaminated with deadly microbes and cancer-causing chemicals. Have I stimulated your appetite - to learn more?

A fowl is a bird of any kind, although some types of birds use the word specifically in their names, like Guinea fowl and Peafowl. Chickens and turkeys are the most popular birds found on people's dinner plates.

In the US, over 35 billion tons of chicken is consumed annually, with a per capita intake of 87 pounds a year. About 18 pounds per person of turkey are consumed each year. The scare of bird flu has had an effect, with chicken consumption down about 90% in European and Indian markets, and chicken prices plummeted.

Besides chicken and turkey, westerners also eat ducks, guinea hens, quail, pheasant's, geese, and ostriches. In other cultures, people are known to eat anything they can catch, including parrots, swans, emus, rheas, and even penguins.

The parts commonly eaten are the muscles, skin, and fat of the fowl. People also eat the heart, liver, and gizzard - collectively known as giblets. A prized delicacy "Foie Gras" (which is French for "fat liver"), is made from the enlarged livers of male ducks and geese. The Chinese even eat the chicken's feet - and chicken feet represented 43% of US poultry sales to China. (Recipe: Wash the chicken feet. Chop off the toenails. The feet are first fried, then marinated, and finally steamed. Yuk!)

Birds as food have traditionally been considered a delicacy - a fare reserved for holidays, like Thanksgiving, or as a treat for Sunday's dinner. Today's practice of "making every day a feast day" has caused a worldwide epidemic of *malnutrition from overnutrition* - now the most important killer of all. Too many calories, and too much fat and protein mean disease - like obesity, heart attacks, cancer, diabetes, arthritis, osteoporosis - and much more suffering.

The fat and protein content of a bird depends in large part upon its diet and activity level. Wild birds are generally much leaner, and therefore lower in fat and higher in protein. *Meat breeds* are chickens developed for their quick growth - heavy with fat and muscle - they are mass-produced specifically to be eaten. The fat and cholesterol in fowl permeate its flesh; they cannot be cut away.

Birds and bird parts with a lower fat content are by nature higher in protein. Excess protein is as damaging to health as is excess fat - causing kidney stones, loss of kidney function, osteoporosis and cancers (lymphomas). You will hardly find a "micro-spec" of dietary fiber or carbohydrate in a dead bird carcass.

Comparison of food values*

Bird (roasted)	Fat % Calories	Protein % Calories	Cholesterol mg/100 Calories
Chicken	51	49	37
Chicken (white meat)	24	76	49
Duck	76	24	25
Goose	65	35	30
Turkey	45	55	40

For Comparison

Beef	50	50	34
Salmon	54	46	31
Potato	01	09	0
Pinto Bean	04	24	0

Note how similar the values of various meats - "a muscle is a muscle..."

Bacteria, viruses, parasites, and fungi found in fowl cause illness and death in humans. The most common pathogens found in commercially processed bird flesh are from their own bowel bacteria and these organisms are Campylobacter, E.coli, and salmonella. During the manufacturing processes used to bring chickens to market, a "fecal soup" is created as thousands of dirty chickens are bathed together. In one study of retail markets in the Washington DC area from June 1999 to July 2000, 70.7% of chicken samples were found to be contaminated with Campylobacter, and 91.1% of the stores visited sold Campylobacter-contaminated chickens. E. coli was found in 38.7% of chicken samples. Approximately 14% of the turkey samples yielded Campylobacter and 11.9% were positive for E. coli. Salmonella was found in 25% of both of these white meats.

Infections with any of these three bacteria can cause symptoms very similar to the flu, like nausea, vomiting, abdominal cramps, diarrhea, fever, chills, weakness, and exhaustion; and can be deadly for children, the elderly, and people with suppressed immune systems. Infections are caused by close contact with the carcasses of birds. Eating the flesh of birds is as close as you can get to their germ-infested tissues. Although cooking destroys most of these infectious agents, people eat, often unknowingly, partially cooked and raw meats.

During the 1997 epidemic of bird flu in Hong Kong, 18 people were infected by contact with birds, resulting in six fatalities. Since then the virus has been spreading from southern China to other parts of the world by migratory birds and, less commonly, by bird trafficking. From December 2003 through March 6, 2006, a total of 175 laboratory-confirmed human avian influenza A (H5N1) infections were reported to WHO from Cambodia, China, Indonesia, Iraq, Thailand, Turkey, and Vietnam. Of these, 95 were fatal. Thus, more than half of the people who get the bird flu die. There is no reliable vaccine for prevention, nor any effective treatment after infection occurs.

In addition to infecting wild birds and poultry, this virus has jumped the species barriers to infect cats, pigs, horses and other mammals. Right now your best strategy is to avoid contact with potentially infected fowl. People traveling abroad are advised, "not to visit birds or poultry farms and markets, to avoid close contact with live or dead poultry and to wash hands often with soap and water". This message means, don't handle (except for your own pets), cook or eat birds.

Whether a bird flu influenza pandemic will occur depends upon whether or not the present viral strains mutate so they can efficiently transfer from humans-to-humans. Influenza A viruses are known for their ease in transforming. Although no human-to-human transmission was documented initially, sporadic cases of such transmission are expected to occur as the infection spreads worldwide. The biological behavior of this virus indicates that once a pandemic begins, isolation of sick people is not likely to contain the spread of disease. A specific vaccine against the bird flu will not be available until six to twelve months after the beginning of the pandemic. This message means that once the disease begins to spread freely among people, you must isolate yourself from the outside world.

Antibiotics are used in the factory-farmed animals to help prevent bird-borne infections and to stimulate growth in order to enhance the profits of the poultry industry. However, heavy use of these drugs hurts people by encouraging the development of antibiotic resistant strains of bacteria. When people become sick they find that the powerful drugs they need have been rendered ineffective. These antibiotics contaminate plants, and are therefore consumed by even the strictest of vegetarians. Manure is used worldwide to grow crops - especially in organic and sustainable agriculture. The antibiotics, like tetracyclines, are completely absorbed by the animal's gut and are then deposited in the animal's feces onto the ground - to be absorbed and incorporated into the growing plants. These drugs present health risks for people who are allergic and become another source for antibiotic-resistant bacteria.

Poultry is high on the food chain. Chemicals from the environment undergo *bioconcentration* when the chickens eat the grains - or worse yet, when chickens are fed pellets containing the remnants of dead cows and/or fishmeal. In these cases the biomagnifications of dangerous chemicals raises levels many hundreds-fold from the original concentration in plants.

The Scenario May Be:

Low concentrations of chemicals are present in the sea vegetables and in the water.

*fish consume these environmental poisons and concentrate them in their body fat;
*cows eat fishmeal and concentrate these noxious wastes even more into their fat;
*then chickens eat dead cow remnants and the toxins become packed further into their flesh;
*finally, people get the strongest doses, as they are at the end of the food chain.

The greatest concentrations of tissue-damaging contaminants are delivered to babies nursing from pollutant-overloaded mothers.

Common Pollutants Found In Poultry

Polycyclic aromatic hydrocarbons (PAHs)
Phthalic acid esters
Polychlorinated dibenzodioxins

Dibenzofurans (PCDDs and PCDFs)
Polychlorinated biphenyls (PCBs)
Organic phosphates

Chicken flesh must be cooked in order to be edible for most humans. The process of cooking chicken flesh leads to the formation of powerful cancer-causing *heterocyclic aromatic amines*. Cooked poultry has some of the highest concentrations of these toxins found in foods commonly consumed. Chickens and turkeys are crowded together in cages barely big enough to allow them to move. Commonly, they are mutilated by cutting off their beaks when they are young. These helpless birds are overstuffed with food and drugs during processing. And finally, their lives are cut short to become food for pets and animals.

People (mostly immigrants) work in dangerous, bloody, greasy surroundings in order to bring fattened fowl to the dinner tables of fattened consumers. AFL-CIO President John J. Sweeney said, "Meat and poultry workers who toil at breakneck speeds in the extremely dangerous and dirty work not only suffer high rates of injuries and deaths but risk losing their jobs when they get hurt, apply for workers' compensation or attempt to improve their lives by trying to form a union."

By showing compassion for tortured animals and underprivileged people working in despicable conditions you will improve the health and well-being of yourself, your family and friends. Everything benefits from enlightened decisions at the dinner table.

References: An article entitled, "How Foul is Fowl"
at www.drmcdougall@drmcdougall.com

Author's note: The bird flu pandemic that never materialized was a scam perpetrated by the pharmaceutical industry to sell vaccines. It was pushed further by the various states' Health Departments. Pimps, Hookers, and Tricks!

Chapter 9

Rumsfeld's Plague: Aspartame!

In a Washington Post article of December 12, 2001, about Donald Rumsfeld, there was a one-liner that was so incredibly relevant. That sentence was: "He could be swilling Diet Coke with the secure knowledge that if not for his turnaround of Big Pharma giant G.D. Searle & Co. and successful touting of the sweetener aspartame, the beverage would not be possible."

If Donald Rumsfeld had never been born, think of how many millions of people the world over would not suffer headaches and dizziness. Thousands blind from the free methyl alcohol in aspartame would have sight, and there would be much fewer cases of optic neuritis and macular degeneration. Millions suffering seizures would live normal lives and wouldn't be taking anti-seizure medication that doesn't work because aspartame interacts with drugs and vaccines. Think of the runner Flo Jo, who drank Diet Coke and died of a grand mal seizure. She, no doubt, would still be alive if she hadn't. Brain fog and memory loss, skyrocketing symptoms of aspartame disease, would not be epidemic.

Millions suffer insomnia because of the depletion of serotonin. Think of Heath Ledger. He took that horrible drug, Ambien CR for sleep, which makes your optic nerve and face swell and give you horrible headaches. Plus, he drank Diet Coke and took other drugs and died of poly-pharmacy. Since aspartame has been proven to be a multi-potential carcinogen, would Farrah Fawcett still be alive?

Consider that constant plague of fallen athletes. Aspartame triggers an irregular heart rhythm and interacts with all cardiac medication. It damages the cardiac conduction system and causes sudden death. Thousands of athletes have fallen. Doctors H.J. Roberts and Russell Blaylock have written many alerts about this.

Epidemiological studies should be done on MS and lupus because of their link to aspartame use. Hundreds of thousands of people suffer from aspartame induced multiple sclerosis and lupus, and if not warned, in time could lose their lives as many have. Hospice nurses have reported Alzheimer's disease in 30-year-olds as it skyrockets from "Rumsfeld's Plague." Think of Michael Jackson, a former Diet Pepsi spokesman. He developed lupus, then came the drugs, then came the serious joint pain and then he died of cardiac arrest which aspartame causes.

As the phenylalanine in aspartame deletes serotonin, it triggers all kinds of psychiatric and behavioral problems. The mental hospitals are full of patients who are nothing more than aspartame victims. If Donald Rumsfeld had never been born, the revoked petition for the approval of aspartame would have been signed by FDA Commissioner Jere Goyan and the mental hospitals would probably house fifty-percent less victims. Jere Goyan would never have been fired at 3:00 AM by the Reagan transition team, in order to overrule the Board of Inquiry. Instead, FDA Commissioner Jere Goyan would have signed the revoked petition into law. FDA today would still be Big Pharma's adversary instead of being their "Hooker".

If aspartame had not been approved, Lou Gehrig's disease, Parkinson's disease and other neuro-degenerative diseases would not be knocking off the public in record numbers. Michael Fox, a Diet Pepsi spokesman, would never have gotten Parkinson's disease at age 30. He would probably still be making movies, young and healthy. Aspartame interacts with L-dopa and other Parkinson drugs. Parcopa has aspartame in it and the pharmaceutical company refuses to remove it.

One has to take a deep breath when you think of how heartless it is that there is not even a warning for pregnant women. Aspartame triggers every kind of birth defect from autism to Tourettes' Syndrome to cleft palate. Aspartame is a drug that induces abortion. As an example, out of 9 pregnancies, 8 were lost and the one that survived is schizophrenic. Multiply that all over the world, due to Rumsfeld's Plague. ADD and ADHD would be rare instead of rampant.

It's normal for young girls to look forward to marriage and children. Yet, many sip on diet soda or use aspartame products not realizing that aspartame is an endocrine disrupting agent, stimulates prolactin, which is a pituitary hormone that stimulates milk production at childbirth, changes the menstrual flow and causes infertility. Many go through life never knowing why they could not have children. Aspartame even destroys marriages because it causes male sexual dysfunction and ruins female response.

Aspartame causes every type of blood disorder from a low blood platelet count to leukemia. Because aspartame can precipitate diabetes, the disease is epidemic. To make matters worse, it can simulate and aggravate diabetic retinopathy and neuropathy, destroy the optic nerve, causes diabetics to go into convulsions and interacts with insulin. Diabetics are losing limbs from the free methyl alcohol and professional organizations like the American Diabetes Association push and defend this poison because they take money from the manufacturers. How many millions would not have diabetes if Rumsfeld had never been born?

Aspartame (NutraSweet/Equal/Spoonful/E951/Candere/Benevia, etc) and MSG, another one of Ajinomoto's horrors, along with their new product Amino Sweet, which is the name they have given to disguise aspartame, are responsible for the epidemic of obesity the world over. Why? Because aspartame makes you crave carbohydrates and causes great toxicity to the liver.

The FDA report lists 92 symptoms from unconsciousness and coma to shortness of breath and shock. Medical texts list even more. See "Aspartame Disease: An Ignored Epidemic", by H.J. Roberts, M.D., and: "Excitotoxins: The Taste That Kills," by neurosurgeon Russell Blaylock, M.D. There is simply no end to the horrors triggered by this literally addictive, excito-neurotoxic, genetically engineered carcinogenic drug. This chemical poison is so deadly that Dr. Bill Deagle, www.nutrimedical.com, a noted Virologist, once said it was worse than depleted uranium because of it being found everywhere in food.

Formaldehyde, which is converted from the free methyl alcohol in aspartame, embalms living tissue and damages DNA according to the Trocho Study done in Barcelona in 1998. Even with his devastating study showing how serious the chemical poison aspartame is, the FDA has turned a blind eye and a deaf ear to it.

With Monsanto attorney Michael Taylor now appointed as deputy to the FDA by President Obama, the FDA is nothing more than Monsanto's Washington Branch Office. Even before the Ramazzini Studies showed aspartame to be a multi-potential carcinogen, the FDA knew it. Their own toxicologist, Dr. Adrian Gross, even admitted that it violated the Delaney Amendment because of the brain tumors and brain cancer. Therefore, no allowable daily intake should ever have been able to be established. Aspartame caused all types of tumors from mammary, uterine, ovarian, pancreatic and thyroid, to testicular and pituitary. Dr. Alemany, who did the Trocho Study, commented that aspartame could kill 200 million people. When you damage DNA you could destroy humanity.

Dr. James Bowen told the FDA over twenty years ago that aspartame is mass poisoning of the American public and more than seventy countries of the world. No wonder it is called, "Rumsfeld's Plague."

Big Pharma knows all about aspartame and they add it to drugs, including the ones used to treat the problems caused by aspartame. Big Pharma has made America a fascist government. People are so sick from aspartame and yet Big Pharma keeps selling these dangerous pharmaceuticals at outrageous prices.

Dr. H.J. Roberts said in one of his books that you have to consider aspartame with killing children. We are talking about a drug that changes brain chemistry. Today, children are medicated instead of educated.

Death and disability is what Donald Rumsfeld has heaped on consumers just to make money. Think of the death of Charles Fleming who used to drink about ten diet sodas a day. Then he used creatine on top of this, which interacts with aspartame and is considered the actual cause of his death. Yet, his wife Diane Fleming, remains in a prison in Virginia convicted of his death, despite being the very one who tried to get her husband to stop using these dangerous products containing aspartame in the first place.

The list and the drama never ends. At least six American Airlines pilots, who were heavy users of aspartame, have died, with one in flight, drinking a Diet Coke. When American Airlines was written about removing aspartame they said, "leave the flying to us." Pilots too, are sick and dying on aspartame, and when you fly, your life is in the hands of the pilot. There was a case where the Delta pilot that died from esophageal cancer had a history of consuming huge quantities of diet sodas. When this was brought to the attention of the Delta management by the pilot's wife, Delta refused her request to alert other pilots.

Then there is the Persian Gulf where diet sodas sat on pallets daily in temperatures ranging from 100° to 120° for as long as nine weeks at a time before the soldiers drank them all day long. Remember, if the methyl alcohol in aspartame converts to formaldehyde at 86° (the body's temperature is 98.6°), it interacts with vaccines, damages the mitochondria or life of the cell, and the whole molecule breaks down to a brain tumor agent.

There is a book out there called, Rumsfeld, His Rise, Fall, and Catastrophic Legacy, by Andrew Cockburn, that will substantiate all of this. And fittingly, Rumsfeld appropriately lives in a place called Mount Misery. In fact, if you would like to contact him with a few kind words, you can at:

Donald Rumsfeld
Mount Misery
23946 Mount Misery Rd.
St. Michael's, MD 21663-2522

In the video, "Sweet Misery: A Poisoned World" (which you can view at my website, www.healthtalkhawaii.com), attorney James Turner explains how Rumsfeld got his poison marketed for human consumption. To learn about how the CDC investigation was covered up in the

Rumsfeld-Pepsi-Nixon connection, go to www.sweetremedy.tv/pages/rumsfeld2.html, or view it in its entirety on my website.

For over a quarter of a century there has been mass poisoning of the public in over 100 countries of the world by aspartame because Donald Rumsfeld, as he puts it, "Called in his markers." The aspartame industry has paid front groups and professional organizations to defend them and push it on the very people to whom it can cause the most harm. A suit was filed against the American Diabetes Association in 2004 for racketeering, but they got out of it.

The hands of physicians are tied. Most are clueless that if the patient is using aspartame, the drugs used to treat the aspartame problem will probably interact and may even contain aspartame. This is the world that Donald Rumsfeld and his plague are responsible for!

My eternal thanks to Dr. Betty Martini, founder of Mission Possible International, for her undying efforts in exposing this heinous crime against humanity and for giving me permission to reprint this article. Dr. Martini's website for all the aspartame information you could ever hope to receive is: www.mpwhi.com.

Chapter 10

Something's "Fishy"

S ince becoming a vegetarian in 1975, I repeatedly hear from health professionals and scientists the suggestion to eat fish to improve health and to reduce the risk of suffering from heart disease. We look at the Japanese as the most recognized example of a fish-eating population that enjoys a low incidence of diseases common to Americans (heart disease, breast cancer, diabetes, etc.), and a trim appearance. Plus, people living in Japan have the longest life expectancy of any country in the world. But maybe these advantages are in spite of the fish, rather than because of the fish. The Japanese are healthy primarily because they eat a diet based on rice with lots of vegetables, and fortunately for them the fish is eaten only as a condiment. But, and there's always a "but", as they adopt the SAD (Standard American Diet), they too experience increased stroke and heart disease.

Okay, let's cut to the chase. Fish is the muscle of a cold-blooded animal with fins and gills. There is no carbohydrate, no dietary fiber, or no vitamin C. Because many fish are high on the food chain they are highly contaminated with environmental chemicals. It is not unusual to read in the newspaper that certain kinds of fish, like swordfish, tuna, or shark, contain sufficient levels of contaminants to be considered a health hazard.

For example, because of their high content of mercury, The Fraud and Drug Administration has advised women who are pregnant or plan to become pregnant, not to eat swordfish, king mackerel, tile fish, shark, or fish from mercury contaminated areas.

Did you know that 60% of the calories of fish comes from fat? And this fat is effortlessly incorporated into a person's body fat, contributing to the risk of obesity. Fish fat is usually associated with a lower risk of cancer. However, there is considerable evidence that the Omega-3 fish fat will increase a person's risk of cancer and will also increase the risk of spreading cancer to other parts of the body. Other unknown facts are that fish fat is known to paralyze the actions of insulin and increase the tendency for high blood sugars and eventually diabetes, and is known to increase the tendency for serious bleeding.

Like all animal products, fish are high in cholesterol. Based on a weight of 100 g, mackerel contains 95 mg of cholesterol, haddock 65 mg, tuna 63 mg, and halibut 50 mg. This compares to beef at 70 mg, chicken at 60 mg, and pork at 70 mg. However, when the comparison is made based on calories, fish (50 mg/100 calories) is much higher in cholesterol than pork (24 mg/100 calories), beef 29 mg/100 calories), or chicken (44 mg/100 calories). Comparisons based upon calories are much more relevant because we eat a diet based on calories (a 2000 calorie diet) rather than based on the weight of the food (a 5 pound diet). Feeding fish to people instead of beef, pork or chicken, causes predictable increases in their blood cholesterol to levels that are virtually identical.

Fish is high in animal protein and the kinds of protein that make up fish are very acidic in nature. The high acid load caused by the ingestion of fish results in bone loss, which eventually leads to osteoporosis. Eskimos are among the highest consumers of fish on earth; they also have the highest rates of osteoporosis of any people on the planet. After the age of 40, Eskimos of both sexes have a 10% to 15% greater bone loss than do Caucasians in the US of the same age. The Eskimos consume up to 2,500 mg of calcium a day, mostly in the form of fish bones. Yet, this large calcium intake is offset by the high protein content (250 to 400 g a day), much of which comes from fish.

I have heard it said that the negative effects of protein on bone health are only caused by synthetic mixtures of proteins devised in the laboratory and are not caused by the real foods that people eat, such as chicken, turkey, beef or fish. The people making the statements failed to thoroughly review the scientific literature and, by no coincidence, most are advocates of high-protein diets.

To support their claim that whole animal foods have no affect on bone loss, they usually quote the work of Herta Spencer from the mid-1970s. She published two often-cited studies on the subject: one, paid for by the National Dairy Council, and the other by the National Livestock and Meat Board. Her work has been rightly criticized because close scrutiny reveals areas of serious inconsistency. For example, in the study paid for by the National Dairy Council, she used inappropriate subjects and reported conclusions in contrast to the results. Of the six subjects in this study, one had osteoporosis and urinary calcium so low as to suggest calcium malabsorption. Another subject carried a diagnosis of hypercalcuria (very high levels of calcium in the urine), making the data invalid. Of the remaining four subjects, three experienced calcium loss during the high-protein diet.

Studies on human subjects using whole foods, such as beef, chicken and turkey have produced negative calcium balances of 77 mg/day. In another study, the addition of 5 ounces of tuna a day (34 g of animal protein) increased the loss of urinary calcium by 23%. Furthermore, scientific evidence shows that the body does not compensate over time while on high-protein diets, and the losses continue for as long as the diet is high in animal protein.

In the United States, between 1983 and 1992, seafood ranks third on the list of products causing food-borne diseases. Several illnesses are a result of toxic algae blooms; for example, the most commonly reported marine toxin disease in the world is ciguatera, associated with consumption of contaminated reef fish such as barracuda, grouper, and snapper. There are about 20,000 cases worldwide. Ciguatera presents primarily as diarrhea, abdominal cramps, vomiting, pain in the teeth, pain on urination, blurred vision, arrhythmias, and heart block. Another common problem from fish is scombroid poisoning. This type of food intoxication is caused by consuming scombroid and scombroid-like marine fish species that have begun to spoil with certain types of bacteria. Fish of the scombroid family are tuna and mackerel.

Fish eat other fish that eat plankton and algae, which are contaminated with environmental pollutants. Because these chemicals are attracted and concentrated in the fat of the fish, they become even more concentrated as the chemicals move up the food chain, by a process known as bio-magnification. The fish most heavily laden with chemicals are those such as the tuna, swordfish and shark, which are predators of smaller sea life.

Unfortunately, those most affected by all this contamination are the ones highest on the food chain - our unborn and breast-feeding children, living off of their mother. PCB exposure of children born to women who had even relatively large quantities of Lake Michigan fish, resulted in poorer intellectual function of the children compared to other children, shown by lower scores on a preschool IQ test, and poorer verbal IQ and reading comprehension at eleven years of age.

Methylmercury is a global environmental problem and is listed as one of the six most dangerous chemicals in the world's environment. An article in the New England Journal of Medicine warned that many fish contain such high levels of mercury that they may actually increase the risk of heart attack. In this study, toenail clippings from men, with a history of previous heart attacks, provided evidence of the person's accumulation of mercury. Those with high mercury levels had more than doubled the risk of a heart attack compared with those who had low levels.

Mercury is known to be toxic to the nervous system and kidneys, but long-term exposure may also accelerate the development of arthrosclerosis by promoting free radical damage to the arteries. Free radicals are highly reactive species of common substances, such as fats and LDL-cholesterol, which donate electrons to tissues and cause severe damage leading to many common diseases. Fish can be a major source of mercury in a very toxic form called methylmercury. This substance may counteract all the hypothesized benefits of Omega-3 fats (fish oil) on prevention of heart disease.

Unless they have been specially processed to remove cholesterol, fish oils contain large amounts of cholesterol and will raise the blood cholesterol of people. Even when the fish oil is purified of cholesterol, the omega-3 fat itself will cause the LDL-bad cholesterol to rise. The final results are published in the study on the effects of fish oil on artery closure, where the authors concluded, "Fish oil treatment for 2 years does not provide favorable changes in the diameter of atherosclerotic coronary arteries."

To get the cholesterol-lowering effects of fish oil you need to consume about 2.5 to 3.5 ounces daily, which represents 675 to 900 extra calories daily. Fish fat is easily stored and to put on an extra five pounds when adding fish oil to a "heart disease prevention program" is a no-brainer. Furthermore, fish oils suppress the immune system, which can promote cancer and increase susceptibility to viral infections, and can cause severe bleeding. Fish fat also inhibits the action of insulin, thus increasing a person's tendency to suffer from diabetes.

So, fish cannot make essential fats because animal systems lack the ability to synthesize omega-3 fats. Seaweeds and algae synthesize these fats that are then stored in the flesh, along with contaminants, cholesterol, animal protein, and calories. To avoid all these hazards, the practical alternative is to simply consume the original source of these "good fats" - plants. The human body has no difficulty converting plant-derived omega-3 fat, alpha linolenic acid, into DHA or other omega-3 fatty acids, supplying all our needs even during gestation and infancy.

The oceans have changed over my 72+-year lifetime. 90% of the large fish - the ones that make baby fish - are gone. 38% of all animal sea life, including blue fin tuna, Atlantic cod, Alaskan King crab, and Pacific salmon have had their populations cut by more than 90%, and 7% of the fish species have become extinct. Because of the rarity of blue fin tuna, the Japanese are now making some of their sushi with beef. The price of fresh wild salmon has increased to $30 a pound, when it's available, which is only a few times a year. Fishing industries have collapsed worldwide and many other coral reefs are now bleached and barren. Reliable predictions warned that by the middle of the century (2048), all fish and seafood species will have collapsed - they will be extinct or on the verge of extinction. The human demand for fish as food has always been the major reason for the devastation of the oceans and part of that demand comes from the belief that fish eating is essential for good health. This is not correct - in fact, in our polluted world, eating fish has become a well-established health hazard.

So because of the cost of fresh wild fish and supposed concerns for the oceans that have been raped and exploited, many people have turned to buying farmed fish. What an interesting concept. What do you do, plant a fish and watch it grow? The problem is that farmed fish is not as idyllic as its concept. Farmed fish are loaded with toxins because they are fed a diet of fish oils and fishmeal obtained from small fish which themselves contain high levels of environmental chemicals. Looking at farmed salmon for example, you will find that they have higher contaminant loads than wild salmon.

Because of the higher cost of meals made with so-called good fats, farmed fish are fed rations containing palm, linseed, rapeseed (a.k.a. canola, which is a GMO), and other cheaper oils. The ultimate fat composition of fish depends upon what they are fed. Therefore, many farmed fish have a balance of fats that would not be considered "heart- healthy."

Other important issues that weigh heavily on the fish farming businesses are the environmental and animal rights. Wastes from fish cages, including doo doo and uneaten food, along with chemicals used in farming, such as pesticides, herbicides, and antibiotics, are dumped into the oceans. When fish and other organisms are kept in close proximity, they breed diseases. In most cases, farmed fish are carnivores, and their feed comes from the ocean; for example, herring is used as salmon feed. Catching herring depletes the food supply for the native fish, including salmon, trout, tuna, grouper, and cod. Also, if you were wondering, fish have feelings too, and life in a fish farm is like living in a prison on death row.

Despite witnessing the first-hand destruction of our environment, we sit back and contribute to its further demise. When I was a kid, the ocean was alive. Now, it's predicted to be dead by the middle of the century. Already, 5000 square miles in the Gulf of Mexico is like the Dead Sea. And British Petroleum did nothing to change that.

For me, fish is not a health food. Since becoming a vegetarian in 1975, I never had concerns about protein, calcium, or the right kind of fats. I just eat a plant-based diet, as organic as humanly possible, minimize my intake of processed foods, and have been fortunate enough to drink non-fluoridated water for the past thirty-five years. And what has that left me with? No illnesses, no medications, and vibrant health. If I can do it, so can you.

References: www.drmcdougall@drmcdougall.com
From Dr. McDougall's articles,
"Fish Is Not Health Food", and
"Confessions Of A Fish Killer"

Chapter 11

MSG: Where You Least Expect It (Opinion)

We all know there is so much controversy regarding MSG. We go to Asian restaurants and automatically say, "no MSG please." Rather than get into the technicalities surrounding the creation of this highly processed chemical substance produced by Ajinomoto, suffice it to say, "If man made it don't eat it."

MSG is a chemical that creates a taste or flavor. It works by making your brain believe that the food you're eating actually tastes good. This in turn means that the manufacturer makes tons of money because they can use crappy products.

Okay let's cut to the chase. A manufacturer would be out of his mind to list MSG as an ingredient. So what they do is to create euphemisms for MSG. So here's what you need to know:

Foods containing these are always MSG:

anything hydrolyzed
anything autolyzed
sodium caseinate

calcium caseinate
textured protein (tvp)
yeast extract
autolyzed yeast
torula yeast

Foods containing these are very likely MSG:

barley malt	anything fortified
malt extract	anything modified
maltodextrin	rice syrup
flavors, flavorings	corn syrup
stock	milk powder
broth	dried milk solids
bouillon	spices
carrageenan	guar gum
whey protein	lecithin (also a GMO)
pectin	enzymes
seasonings	soy protein

In addition to the horrors of aspartame if you have something that's bothering you and your doctor can't put his finger on it, chances are there's a good chance of it being MSG related.

Short and sweet: read labels, read labels, read labels! And above all, like I said, IF MAN MADE IT, DON'T EAT IT.

If you're not convinced and need more documentation go check out books by Dr. Russell Blaylock (Excitotoxins:The Taste That Kills).

Bear in mind that most doctors are clueless about the toxic effects of MSG. In addition, because of the enormous amount of money generated by the MSG industry, MSG producers and lobbyists will do their best to make you believe that it is safe. If you have processed foods in your diet you are getting a steady dose of MSG. So the solution is quite simple. If you want to avoid MSG, it is best to avoid processed foods, canned foods, boxed foods, or commercially prepared foods.

Trust me, in the beginning you may think it's a pain in the butt to prepare all your food from scratch. However, it sure beats the ramifications of this synthetic chemical poison.

Chapter 12

The Sugar Conspiracy

With the food industry, it all comes down to greed and various conspiracies to make you eat and spend more. As their profits go through the roof, every time you use more of their products, you need to realize that they are already producing enough food for every American to eat 3,900 calories a day - which is almost double what we actually need. So, how do they get us to eat more girth-enlarging calories? Sugar!

Sugar and corn sweetener, affectionately known as high fructose corn syrup and soon *corn sugar*, aside from being largely a GMO crop, are cheap to produce and let you eat until the cows come home without feeling full. To scarf down 1,000 calories via a fountain drink at the local convenience store is not only effortless, but it leaves plenty of room for dinner.

The effect is that this type of consumption has you eat more calories than your body needs; you easily gain weight; and it's easier to become the President than to lose weight.

We, the "Tricks," are eating what amounts to 31 teaspoons of added sugar a day, which equates to about 500 extra calories a day, or 25% of your daily caloric intake each and every day.

So, how do they trick us into doing that?

The "Hooker" (the U.S. Government) requires that the "Pimp" (the food industry) disclose the amount of sugar contained in a given product. Sounds great on paper, doesn't it?

What if sugar had a different name, one that you may not be aware of? Having somewhat of a brain, you would assume that molasses and honey must contain sugar. But what about sorghum, or corn syrup, or high fructose corn syrup, or turbinado, or amazake, or fructose, or lactose, or dextrose, or sucrose, or galactose, or maltose? It's enough to make you comatose!

The average person wouldn't associate these scientific-sounding names with sugar. But that's what they are. The sugar aliases allow a food manufacturer to list these euphemisms on the same label without telling you it's all sugar. The next trick they use is to list the information in grams. Why grams? Because most people don't know squat about grams!

When you see that a 12-ounce can of soda contains 40g of sugar, you could care less. But what if you saw that that same can of soda contains 10 teaspoons of sugar? What would you think if you were sitting next to a guy in a restaurant and you watched him put 10 teaspoons of sugar in his coffee? You would think the guy was lolo (Hawaiian for crazy), wouldn't you?

So this will make it easy for you. Four grams equals one teaspoon. You divide the total grams by four, you will know how many teaspoons of sugar you are about to ingest.

One very, very important thing to remember is that you must read labels because many "non-sweetened" products contain sugar as well. A half-cup of store-bought spaghetti sauce can contain as much as three teaspoons of sugar. Ketchup can have a 20% sugar content.

When the "Pimps" take the fat out of a product, like cookies or salad dressing, guess what they replace it with? Yep, sugar and extra salt. High blood pressure anyone? Calorie-wise, they are not much less than the fattier version. Bread is another one. It is sugar and eggs. White sugar, by the way, is used in aircraft paint because it doesn't crack under extreme temperatures. It is what gives bread its nice, golden crust.

We know that potato chips are salty, but they contain sugar as well. They don't say, "betcha can't eat just one," for nothing. And let's not forget the popular high-protein energy bars. These guys can contain up to 300 calories and are loaded with sugar.

There was a study done at the American College of Neuropsycho-pharmacology (say that three times fast and you'll own it), which found that sugar gives the same brain reaction as morphine, cocaine, and nicotine. To put it another way, sugar is addictive!

The reality is that the food industry knows full well that sugar is addictive, so it shouldn't come as a surprise to you that they will put as much as they can in as many products as they can to get you to eat more and more and more. You eat more, you get fat, you get sick, they get rich. They see that as a win-win situation. How do you see it?

But sugar just doesn't make you waddle down the street. It does a number on your insulin levels and leads you to becoming a diabetic. Did you know that just consuming one can of soda a day increases your risk of diabetes by 85% and can cut eleven to twenty years off of your life?

It's not a walk in the park to break the sugar habit, but you have to give it your best shot. You can keep your blood sugar stable by including protein with every meal. If you know about quinoa, the incredible grain from Peru, which is a complete protein, you can eat that and get plenty of fiber as well. Remember, if it had a face or a mother, it has no fiber.

If you use fruit as a substitute for sugar it will help curtail your sugar cravings. And, under no circumstances, substitute fake sugar and think it's the answer. Aspartame will turn you into a zombie because the methanol in aspartame converts to formaldehyde at 84°F (the body's temperature is 98.6°F). Sucralose, aka Splenda, is derived from chlorine and is best used in your swimming pool. The reality is that these fake sugars do not eliminate sugar cravings, they actually increase them. A study proved that a person's risk for obesity went up 41% for each daily can of diet soda.

So, do the best you can and take it one day at a time. When you see your weight come down and your mood swings level out and you have more sustained energy, you'll know you're on the right road. But when push comes to shove, just stay as sweet as you *naturally* are.

Chapter 13

"Dem Bones, Dem Bones,
Dem Dry Bones"

Muscle, vitality, strength, power, energy, vigor, aggressiveness, and liveliness are words that come to mind when people think of the benefits of protein in their diet. The truth is quite the opposite. Bone loss, osteoporosis, kidney damage, immune dysfunction, arthritis, cancer promotion, low energy, and overall poor health are the real consequences from over emphasizing protein.

Protein serves as raw material to build tissues. Without sufficient protein from your diet, your body would be in trouble. But, aside from starvation, this never happens. Yes, a little protein is good, but more is not better. Protein consumed beyond our needs is a health hazard as devastating as excess dietary fat and cholesterol. Unfortunately, almost everyone on the typical western diet is overburdened with protein to the point of physical collapse. The public has almost no awareness of problems of protein overload, but scientists have known about the damaging effects of excess protein for more than a century.

In his book, _Physiology Economy in Nutrition_, Russell Henry Chittenden, former President of the American Physiological Society and Professor of Physiological Chemistry at Yale University, wrote in 1905, "Proteid (protein) decomposition products are a constant menace to the well-being of the body; any quantity of proteid or albuminous food beyond the real requirements of the body may prove distinctly injurious... Further, it requires no imagination to understand the constant strain upon the liver and kidneys, to say nothing of the possible influence upon the central and peripheral parts of the nervous system by those nitrogenous waste products which the body ordinarily gets rid of as speedily as possible."

Let's take an analogy. Say you were building a house that requires 100 sheets of plywood, but the lumberyard delivers 200 sheets. Initially, you might think this is a good thing - a real windfall. But what do you really have? A big pile of expensive lumber cluttering your yard. The mass is an eyesore, a fire hazard, a potential source of physical injury, and it detracts from your property value. Disposal of the excess lumber will be costly and could result in physical injury. To make matters worse, the lumberyard delivered "Fire Retardant Treated" plywood. The fire retardants used are very acidic, and under humid conditions the acids weaken the lumber, leading to a potential structural failure of your house - a catastrophic threat to life and limb - not to mention your pocketbook. The lesson learned here is when building a house, take delivery of only the amount of lumber you actually need - and use only the safest construction materials.

What then, are your construction (protein) needs? Protein from your diet is required to build new cells, synthesize hormones, and repair damaged and worn out tissues. So, how much do you need?

The protein loss from the body each day from shedding skin, sloughing intestine, and other miscellaneous losses is about 3 g per day. Add to this loss other physiological requirements, such as growth and repairs. The final tally, based on solid scientific research is, "**Your total daily need for protein is about 20 to 30 grams.**" Plant proteins easily meet these needs.

So what are people consuming? Those living in many rural Asian societies consume about 40 to 60 g from their diet of starch (mostly rice) with vegetables. On the Western diet, typical food choices centered around meat and dairy products, "a well-balanced diet," provides about 100 to 160 g of protein a day. A traditional Eskimo, eating marine animals, or someone on the Atkins diet with various kinds of meat and dairy, might be consuming 200 to 400 g a day. Notice that there can be a ten-fold (1000%) difference from our basic requirements and the amount some people consume. The resilience of the human body allows for survival under conditions of incredible over-consumption.

Once the body's needs are met, then the excess must be removed. The liver converts the excess protein into urea and other nitrogen-containing breakdown products, which are finally eliminated through the kidneys as part of the urine.

Processing all that excess dietary protein - as much as 300 g (10 ounces) a day - causes wear and tear on the kidneys. As a result, on average, 25% of kidney function is lost over a lifetime (70 years) from consuming the western diet.

Fortunately, the kidneys are built with large reserve capacity and the effects of losing one quarter of kidney function are of no consequence for otherwise healthy people. However, people who have already lost kidney function for other reasons - from an accident, donation of the kidney, infection, diabetes, and hypertension - may suffer life-threatening consequences from a diet no higher in protein than the average American consumes.

The time-honored fundamental treatment for people with failing kidneys is a low-protein diet. End-stage kidney failure, requiring dialysis, can usually be postponed or avoided by patients fortunate enough to learn about the benefits of a low-protein diet.

People suffering with liver failure are also placed on diets low in protein as fundamental therapy - short of a liver transplant this is the most important therapy they will receive. During the end stages of liver failure, patients will often fall into a coma from the build-up of protein breakdown products (hepatic coma). A change to a cost-free, very low-protein diet can cause these dying people to awaken. Well-planned, plant-food-based diets are particularly effective with both kidney and liver disease.

Worldwide, rates of hip fractures and kidney stones increase with increasing animal protein consumption, including dairy products. For example, people from the USA, Canada, Norway, Sweden, Australia and New Zealand have the highest rates of osteoporosis. The lowest rates are among people who eat the fewest animal-derived foods (these people are also on lower calcium diets) - like the people from rural Asia and rural Africa.

Osteoporosis is caused by several controllable factors; however, the most important one is the foods we choose - especially the amount of animal protein and the foods high in acid. The high-acid foods are meat, poultry, fish, seafood, and hard cheeses - parmesan cheese is the most acidic of all foods commonly consumed. This acid must be neutralized by the body. Carbonate, citrate and sodium are alkaline materials released from the bones to neutralize the acids. Fruits and vegetables are alkaline and as a result a diet high in these plant foods will neutralize acid and preserve bones. The acidic condition of the body caused by the western diet also raises cortisol (steroid) levels. Elevated cortisol causes severe chronic bone loss - just like giving steroid medication for arthritis causes severe osteoporosis.

Let's compare the acid load of various foods, indicating the renal acid load per 100 calories. Bear in mind that a positive value indicates acidic, where a negative value indicates alkaline.

Beef	6.3
Chicken	7.0
Fish	9.3
Cheddar Cheese	10.0
Potato	-5.0
Peas	1.0
Wheat Flour	1.0
Banana	-6.0
Apple	-5.0
Spinach	-56.0
Tomato	-18.0

Once materials are released from the solid bone, the calcium and other bone substances move through the bloodstream to the kidneys where they are eliminated in the urine. In an effort to remove the overabundance of waste protein, the flow of blood to the kidneys increases - the result: calcium is filtered out of the body. Naturally, the kidneys attempt to return much of this filtered calcium back to the body; unfortunately, the acid and sulfur-containing amino acids from the animal foods thwart the body's attempts to conserve calcium. As a result each 10 g of dietary protein in excess of our needs (30 g daily) increases daily urinary calcium loss by 16 mg. Another way of looking at the effects are: doubling dietary protein intake increases the loss of calcium in our urine by 50%. Plant proteins (plant-food based) do not have these calcium and bone- losing effects under normal living conditions.

Once this bone material arrives in the collecting systems of the kidney it easily precipitates into solid formations known as kidney stones. Over 90% of kidney stones found in people following a high-protein, western diet are formed primarily of bone-derived calcium. Following a healthy diet is the best way to prevent kidney stones.

The qualities of the proteins we consume are as important as the quantities. One very important distinction between animal and plant-derived protein is that animal proteins contain very large amounts of the basic element *sulfur.* This sulfur is found as two of the 20 primary amino acids, *methionine* and *cysteine.* Derived from these two primary sulfur-containing amino acids are several other sulfur-containing amino acids: keto-methionine, cystine, homocysteine, cystathionine, taurine, and cysteic acid.

Comparing the relative amounts of the sulfur-containing amino acid, methionine, found in the following foods, based on the same number of calories, we find that:

   *Beef provides four times more than pinto beans
   *Eggs have four times more than corn
   *Cheddar cheese has five times more than white potatoes
   *Chicken provides seven times more than rice
   *Tuna provides twelve times more than sweet potatoes

Even though sulfur-containing amino acids are essential for our survival, an excess of these amino acids beyond our needs places a critical burden upon our body and detracts from our health in six important ways:

1) Amino acids, as the name implies, are acids; the sulfur-containing amino acids are the strongest acids of all as they break down into powerful *sulfuric acid.* Excess acid, as discussed above, is a primary cause of bone loss leading to osteoporosis and kidney stone formation.

2) Methionine is metabolized into homocysteine. Animal foods are the major source of the amino acid, homocysteine, in people. The more meat in the diet, the higher a person's blood level of homocysteine. A diet high in fruits and vegetables lowers the levels of this amino acid. Epidemiological and clinical studies have proven homocysteine to be an independent risk factor for heart attacks, strokes, closure of the arteries to the legs, (peripheral vascular disease), blood clots in the legs (venous thrombosis), thinking problems (cognitive impairment), and even worse mental troubles, like dementia, Alzheimer's disease, and depression.

3) Sulfur feeds cancerous tumors. Cancerous cell metabolism is dependent upon methionine being in the diet; whereas, normal cells can grow on a methionine-free diet (feeding off other sulfur-containing amino acids). This methionine dependency has been demonstrated for breast, lung, colon, kidney, melanoma, and brain cancers. Increasing methionine in the diet of animals promotes the growth of cancer.

There is also evidence of cancer-promoting effects of methionine medicated through a powerful growth stimulating hormone called, *insulin-like growth factor - 1* (IGF-1). Meat and dairy products raise IGF-1 levels and promote the growth of cancers of the breast, colon, prostate, and lung.

4) Sulfur from sulfur-containing amino acids is known to be toxic to the tissues of the intestine, and to have deleterious effects on the human colon, even at low levels. The consequence of a diet of high-methionine (animal) foods may be a life-threatening inflammatory bowel disease, called ulcerative colitis.

5) Sulfur restriction prolongs life. Almost eighty years ago, restricting food consumption was found to prolong the life of animals by changing the fundamental rate at which aging occurs. Restriction of methionine in the diet has also been shown to prolong the life of experimental animals. By no coincidence, a diet based on plant foods is inherently low in both calories and methionine - thus the easiest and most effective means to a long and healthy life.

6) Possibly a stronger motivation to keep protein, and especially methionine-rich animal protein, out of your diet is foul smelling odors - halitosis, body odor, and stinky farts - akin to the smell of rotten eggs - are direct results of the sulfur (animal protein) you eat.

Animal foods, full of protein waste, promote poor health and early death by accelerating the aging process and increasing the risk of diseases, like heart disease, diabetes, and cancer, that in their own right, cause premature death. From now on, think of the excess protein you consume **as garbage** that must be disposed of in order to avoid toxic waste accumulation. Obviously, the best action is to avoid the excess in the first place and this is most easily accomplished by choosing a diet based on starches, vegetables, and fruits. Within a few days of changing to a healthy diet, most of the waste will be gone and the damaged tissues will begin healing.

Unfortunately, you will find little support for such an obvious, inexpensive, and scientifically-supported approach - especially when the common masses of people worldwide are ignorant of the truth. Most are gobbling down as much protein as they can stuff in their mouths and the food industry is supporting this behavior by advertising their products as "high-protein" and "Atkins-approved" (Dr. Atkins dropped dead of a heart attack on the sidewalk in New York City) - as if this was somehow good for the body. The paradox is age-old, and because it is ruled by emotions rather than by clear thinking, a change in mind-set in your lifetime should be expected.

Two thousand years ago, in this Bible passage, Paul asked for tolerance between meat eaters and vegetarians (Romans 14: 1-2). "One man's faith allows him to eat everything, but another man, whose faith is weak, eats only vegetables. The man who eats everything must not look down on him who does not, and the man who does not eat everything must not condemn the man who does... "Do not wait for consensus before you take action."

As Obama says: "The time for change is now."

Reprinted with permission (and modification) by Dr. John McDougall, from his article, "Protein Overload", found on his website @ www. drmcdougall@drmcdougall.com

Chapter 14

Calcium Deposits

When you tell someone you're a vegetarian or vegan, invariably the first question you're asked is, "How do you get your protein?" Well, the answer to that question has been answered in a previous chapter. The second question you likely get is, "If you don't eat dairy products, how do you get your calcium?"

In answering this question the best way to answer it is in the form of questions and answers. The questions are questions that people would normally ask and we'll leave that up to many reliable sources like physicians, dietitians, and researchers to supply the answers.

Q: What is calcium?

A: "Calcium is a mineral that the body needs for numerous functions, including building and maintaining bones and teeth, blood clotting, the transmission of nerve impulses, and the regulation of the heart's rhythm. Ninety-nine percent of the calcium in the human body is stored in the bones and teeth. The remaining 1% is found in the blood and other tissues."

Source: Harvard School of Public Health

Q: How does the body acquire calcium?

A: "The body gets the calcium it needs in two ways. One, is by eating foods that contain calcium. Good sources include dairy products, which have the highest concentration per serving of highly absorbable calcium, and dark leafy greens or dried beans, which have varying amounts of absorbable calcium."

"The other way the body gets calcium is by pulling it from the bones. This happens when the blood levels of calcium drop too low, usually when it's been a while since having eaten a meal containing calcium. Ideally, the calcium that is "borrowed" from the bones will be replaced at a later point. But, this doesn't always happen. Most important, this payback cannot be accomplished simply by eating more calcium."

Source: Harvard School of Public Health

Q: How much calcium do I need?

A: according to the Office of Dietary Supplements of the National Institutes of Health, the amount needed varies by age group but not by sex. The following chart depicts their recommendations:

Recommended Calcium Adequate intake

Male and Female Age	Calcium (mg per day)
0 to 6 months	210
7 to 12 months	270
1 to 3 years	500
4 to 8 years	800
9 to 13 years	1300
14 to 18 years	1300
19 to 50 years	1000
51+ years	1200
Pregnant/Lactating Women	1000

Source: Office of Dietary Supplements, NIH Clinical Center, National Institute of Health

Dr. John McDougall takes a different view. He writes, "Studies have shown that an intake of 150 to 200 mg of calcium daily is adequate to meet the needs of most people, even during pregnancy and lactation. And in fact, most of the world's population ingests 300 to 500 mg of calcium each day. Calcium is so efficiently absorbed by the human intestine and so sufficient in diets of mankind, that calcium deficiency of dietary origin is unknown in human beings.

"Only in those places where calcium and protein are eaten in relatively high quantities does a deficiency of bone calcium exist at such epidemic rates, due to an excess of animal protein."

Source: *The McDougall Program for a healthy heart, 256*

Q: Are most Americans meeting the recommended intake for calcium?

A: according to a Continuing Survey of Food intakes of Individuals conducted by the US Department of Agriculture between the years 1994 and 1996, the following percentage of Americans did not meet the recommended intake for calcium;
    *44% of boys and 58% of girls ages 6 to 11
    *64% of boys and 87% of girls ages 12 to 19
    *55% of men and 78% of women ages 20+

Source: Office of Dietary Supplements, NIH Clinical Center, National Institutes of Health

Q: How can I recognize if I am deficient in calcium?

A: Dr. Holly Roberts says, "If you have a calcium deficiency, you may develop twitching, nerve sensitivity, brittle nails, insomnia, depression, numbness, and heart palpitations. Painful muscle cramps in the calves may occur often during pregnancy, particularly in women who are deficient in calcium."

Source: *Your Vegetarian Pregnancy, 111*

Q: Are dairy products the best source of calcium?

A: Dr. Walter Willett says, "Milk is clearly the most efficient way to get calcium from food, since it delivers almost 300 mg per eight-ounce glass.

Few other foods come close to packing in that much calcium. But milk delivers more than just calcium, and some of its other components, like extra calories, saturated fat, and sugar known as galactose, aren't necessarily good for you. What's more, as many as 50 million adults in the United States cannot completely digest the milk sugar known as lactose nor can most of the world's population".

"Dairy products should not occupy the prominent place that they do in the USDA Pyramid, nor should they be the centerpiece of the national strategy to prevent osteoporosis. Instead, the evidence shows that dietary calcium should come from a variety of sources and, if more calcium is really needed, from cheap, no calorie, easy to take supplements. Then you can look at dairy products as an optional part of a healthy diet and take them in moderation, if at all."

Source: *Eat, Drink, and Be Healthy*, 139

Dr. Willett adds, "If no one really knows the best daily calcium target, then why not play it safe and boost your calcium by drinking three glasses a day? Here are five good reasons: lactose intolerance, saturated fat, extra calories, a possible increased risk of prostate cancer, and a possible increased risk of ovarian cancer."

Source: *Eat, Drink, and Be Healthy*, 144

Dr. Neal Barnhard writes, "Dairy products contain sex hormones, too. Farmers keep dairy cattle pregnant virtually constantly. This keeps their milk production high. The hormones circulating in a pregnant cow's blood easily passes into her milk. In fact, one of the ways farmers test whether their cows are pregnant or not is to measure estrogens in their milk. You cannot taste them, but they are there. These hormones end up in milk regardless of whether the farmer gives extra hormones to the cow; the cow makes them herself and they go straight into her milk. Several population studies have shown a correlation between dairy product consumption and breast cancer incidence."

Source: *Eat Right, Live Longer*, 71-72

Q: Will consuming dairy products protect me from developing osteoporosis?

A: Dr. Joel Fuhrman says, "Hip fractures and osteoporosis are more frequent in populations in which dairy products are commonly consumed and calcium intakes are commonly high. For example, American women drink 30 to 32 times as much cow's milk as the New Guineans, yet suffer 47 times as many broken hips. A multi-country analysis of hip fracture incidence and dairy product consumption found that milk consumption has a high statistical association with higher rates of hip fractures."

Source: _Eat to Live_, 84

Dr. T. Colin Campbell says: "Americans consume more cow's milk and its products per person than most populations in the world. So Americans should have wonderfully strong bones, right? Unfortunately not. A recent study showed that American women aged 50 and older have one of the highest rates of hip fractures in the world. The only countries with higher rates are in Europe and in the South Pacific (Australia and New Zealand) where they consume even more milk than the United States."

Source: _The China Study_, 204

Dr. Fuhrman states, "There are many good reasons not to consume dairy. For example, there was a strong association between the dairy lactose and ischemic heart disease. There was also a clear association between high-growth-promoting foods such as dairy products and cancer. There is a clear association between milk consumption and testicular cancer. Dairy fat is also loaded with various toxins and is the primary source of our nation's high exposure to dioxin. Dioxin is a highly toxic chemical compound that even the U.S. Environmental Protection Agency admits is a prominent cause of many types of cancer in those consuming dairy fat, such as butter and cheese. Cheese is also a power inducer of acid load, which increases calcium loss further. Considering that cheese and butter are the foods with the highest saturated fat content and a major source of our dioxin exposure, cheese is a particularly foolish choice for obtaining calcium".

Source: _Eat to Live_, 88-89

Q: What role does phosphorous play in calcium deficiency?

A: Dr. Holly Roberts says, "Calcium deficiency can occur, not only if your diet is low in calcium, but also if your diet is high in phosphorus. The ratio of calcium and phosphorus in your bones it's 2.5 to 1. If your diet includes higher levels of calcium then phosphorus, it is more likely that you will maintain this healthy ratio and healthy bones. To do this, it is best if you maintain a ratio of phosphorous to calcium within your diet of 1:1. The diet of many Americans contains a phosphorus-to-calcium ratio 4:1. Calcium is a positive ion, which means they will bind with negative ions. Foods that contain phosphorus form negative ions. So if you have excess phosphorus in your diet, it will bind calcium to it and you will excrete both of these minerals. If such a situation develops, you may actually lose more calcium than you took in, and you will deplete the calcium stored in your bones. Phosphorus is present in carbonated drinks, meat, eggs, and cheese spreads".

"You will absorb higher levels of calcium if your diet contains adequate amounts of vitamin D, magnesium, dairy products, and vitamin C. Regular exercise helps the body absorb calcium. However, if you follow a high-fat or high-protein diet that is rich in phosphorus, it will be more difficult for your body to absorb calcium."

Source: _Your Vegetarian Pregnancy_, 111

Q: What happens if I get too much calcium?

A: The Linus Pauling Institute at Oregon State University states, "Abnormally elevated blood calcium (hypercalcemia) resulting from the over consumption of calcium has never been documented to occur from foods, only from calcium supplements. Mild hypercalcemia may be without symptoms, or may result in the loss of appetite, nausea, vomiting, constipation, abdominal pain, dry mouth, thirst, and frequent urination. More severe hypercalcemia may result in confusion, delirium, coma, and if not treated, death. Hypercalcemia has been reported only with the consumption of high quantities of calcium supplements usually in combination with antacids, particularly in the days when peptic ulcers were treated with large quantities of milk, calcium carbonate (antacid) and sodium bicarbonate (absorbable alkali). The condition was termed _milk alkali syndrome,_ and has been reported at calcium supplement levels from 1.5 to 16.5 grams per day for 2 days to 30 years. Since the treatment for peptic ulcers has changed, the incidence of this syndrome has decreased considerably".

Source: *"Calcium"*. Linus Pauling Institute at Oregon State University.

Q: if I follow a vegan diet, do I need as much calcium as people on the Standard American Diet?

A: Registered dietitians Vesanto Melina and Brenda Davis write:

Adequate Intakes Of Calcium For Adults

Age	AI Calcium mg
19-50 years	1000
Over 50 years	1200

"Because calcium needs are influenced by a host of factors, it is extremely difficult for nutrition experts to determine exactly how much calcium an individual needs to function at optimum levels and to continue into old age with healthy, strong bones. In fact, it has been such a challenge that the recommendations are now called,' Adequate Intakes' (AI) and are a sort of 'best guess', used when there is insufficient data to make a firm recommendation. These 'Adequate Intakes' may seem high. Remember, that they are based on the needs of the general North American population, with high amounts of sodium and meat-centered diets providing much more protein than needed. To make things worse, the population is largely sedentary, a factor that works against the retention of minerals in bones."

"It is possible that the calcium requirements of vegans and of other vegetarians are lower in the general population, particularly if:

*protein intakes are adequate and yet closer to recommendations
*sodium intake is not over 2400 mg/day, on average
*there is regular participation in weight-bearing exercise.

"However, note that salt, tamari, and miso are vegan food ingredients. Though plant proteins are somewhat lower in sulfur-containing amino acids, vegans should not assume they are protected from osteoporosis because of lower protein intakes."

Source: *Becoming Vegan*, 95

Q: How much calcium do we absorb from the foods we eat?

A: Melina and Davis point out, "On average, North Americans absorb about 30% of the calcium that is present in our diets, but when you take into account the amounts lost in urine and feces, the actual amount we *retain* may be as low as 10% of what was in our food. From the calcium that makes its way into our bodies, there can be substantial losses, depending on certain characteristics of our diet, particularly the protein and sodium contents. A single fast food hamburger could result in calcium losses of about 23 mg. However, if we retain only 10% of what was in our diet, that burger would, in effect, increase dietary calcium needs by 230 mg."

Source: *Becoming Vegan*, 93

Dr. John McDougall says: "Humans have a highly efficient intestinal tract that, under almost every circumstance, will absorb the correct amount of calcium to meet the body's needs. The intestinal cells act as regulators for the amount of calcium that enters the body. When the calcium content of the diet is low, a relatively higher percentage of calcium will be absorbed from the foods. If the diet is high in calcium, a smaller percentage of the calcium will be absorbed but the body's need is always the controlling factor regulating the entry of calcium into the cells of the intestinal wall."

Source: *The McDougall Program for a Healthy Heart*, 255-256

Q: What triggers the body to pull calcium from the bones?

A: Dr. Fuhrman provides the following list:

Dietary Factors That Induce Calcium Loss in the Urine

animal protein
salt
caffeine
refined sugar

alcohol
nicotine
aluminum-containing antacids
drugs such as antibiotics, steroids, thyroid hormone
vitamin A supplements
Source: _Eat to Live_, 86

Dr. Neal Barnard provides his list:

Calcium Depleters

animal protein
caffeine
excess phosphorus (sodas, animal products)
sodium (animal products, canned or snack foods)
tobacco
sedentary lifestyle

Source: _Eat Right, Live Longer_, 167

Davis and Melina say, "When the kidneys excrete excess sodium, 23 to 26 mg of calcium is lost along with every gram of sodium excreted".

Source: _Becoming Vegan_, 94

Q: Why is a vegetarian diet better for bone health?

A: Dr. Neil Barnard explains: " A meat-based diet is disastrous for bones. Switching from beef to chicken or fish does not help because these products have as much animal protein as beef or even a bit more. Bodybuilders and others who take protein supplements have even greater calcium losses. The problem is not just the amount of protein in meats but also the type. Meats are loaded with what are called sulfur-containing amino acids, which are especially aggressive at causing calcium to be lost in the urine."

Source: _Eat Right, Live Longer_, 162-163

In looking at calcium loss, Dr. Joel Fuhrman states, "Published data clearly links increased urinary excretion of calcium with animal-protein intake but not with vegetable-protein intake. Plant foods, though some may be high in protein, are not acid-forming. Animal-protein ingestion results in a heavy acid load in the blood. This sets off a series of reactions whereby calcium is released from the bones to help neutralize the acid. The sulfur-based amino acids in animal products contribute significantly to urinary acid production in the resulting calcium loss. The Nurses Health Study found that women who consumed 95 g of protein a day had a 22% greater risk of forearm fracture than those who consumed less than 68 g."

Source: *Eat To Live*, 86

Dr. Dean Ornish says, "The real cause of osteoporosis in this country is not insufficient calcium intake, it is excessive excretion of calcium in the urine. Even calcium supplementation is often not enough to make up for the increased calcium excretion. Vegetarians, in contrast, excrete much less calcium, and this is why they have very low rates of osteoporosis even though their dietary intake of calcium is lower than those on the meat-eating diet."

Source: *Dr. Dean Ornish's Program For Reversing Heart Disease*, 301

Q: What are good food sources for calcium?

A: "Dairy products are not the healthiest source," says Dr. Neal Barnard. "They too contain calcium, but only about 30% of it is absorbed. The remaining 70% never makes it past the intestinal wall and is simply excreted with the feces. Dairy products have many other undesirable features, including animal proteins that contribute in some cases, to arthritis and respiratory problems, lactose sugar that is linked to cataracts, frequent traces of antibiotics, and other problems that lead many doctors to suggest that we avoid them and get calcium from healthier sources.

"The healthiest calcium sources are 'greens and beans'. Green leafy vegetables are loaded with calcium. One cup of broccoli has 178 mg of calcium. What's more, the calcium in broccoli and most other green leafy vegetables is more absorbable then the calcium in milk. An exception is spinach, which has a form of calcium that is not well absorbed.

"Beans, lentils and other legumes are also loaded with calcium. We think of beans as a humble food, but they are an extraordinary source of nutrition. They have calcium, omega-3 fatty acids, the cholesterol-lowering soluble fiber that many people thought was only in oat bran, and healthy complex carbohydrates. If you make green vegetables and beans regular parts of your diet, you'll get two excellent sources of calcium."

Source: *Eat Right, Live Longer,* 168

Dr. Fuhrman agrees by writing, "You do not need dairy products to get sufficient calcium if you lead a healthy diet. All unprocessed natural foods are calcium-rich; even a whole orange (not orange juice) has about 60 mg of calcium."

Source: *Eat To Live,* 80-90

Dr. John McDougall says, "A vegetable-based diet is rich in calcium and all the other nutrients the body needs. Let's not forget that the original source of all calcium is the earth, and plants make this mineral available to animals, including humans, in delicious, digestible packages. That's where all the animals get it from and you can too."

Source: *The McDougall Program for a Healthy Heart,* 256

Q: What role does vitamin D play in relation to calcium?

A: In *Becoming Vegan,* the authors write, "Vitamin D is a major player in a team of nutrients and hormones that keep blood calcium at optimum levels in supporting bone health during growth and throughout life. It stimulates the absorption of the bone-building minerals calcium and phosphorus from the intestine and helps regulate the amount of calcium and bone. It is important for proper functioning of cells throughout the body (in muscle, nerves, and glands) that depend on calcium. If more blood calcium is needed, vitamin D is able to act in three places:
   1. To reduce urinary calcium losses via the kidneys;
   2. To absorb calcium from food more efficiently in the digestive tract;
   3. To draw calcium from our bones, which serve as a storehouse of calcium."

Source: *Becoming Vegan,* 133-134

Q: How is vitamin K related to calcium?

A: Dr. Walter Willett writes, "Until recently, vitamin K was thought to be necessary mostly for the formation of proteins that regulate blood clotting.

It turns out, though, that this fat-soluble vitamin also plays one or more roles in the regulation of calcium and the formation and stabilization of bone. So, too little vitamin K may help set the stage for osteoporosis. In the Nurses' Health Study, women who got more than 109 mcg vitamin K a day were 30% less likely to break a hip than women who got less than that amount. Vitamin K is mainly found in green vegetables such as dark green lettuce, broccoli, spinach, Brussels sprouts, and kale. Eating one or more servings of these foods a day should give you enough vitamin K."

Source: _Eat, Drink, and Be Healthy_, 150

About the Experts:

Dr. Charles R. Attwood (deceased) was a board-certified pediatrician and Fellow of the American Academy of Pediatrics. He practiced medicine for 35 years - first in San Francisco, and then in Crowley, Louisiana. He is the author of _Dr Attwood's Low-Fat Prescription For Kids_ and wrote hundreds of newspaper articles on the health effects of nutrition and fitness. Dr. Attwood co-authored a regular column with Dr. Benjamin Spock in the nationally respected publication, _New Century Nutrition_, and worked as a consultant with Dr. Spock to revise the nutrition sections of the classic, _Dr. Spock's Baby and Child Care_. He was selected as a faculty member of the American Academy of Nutrition and was a guest lecturer at Cornell University.

Dr. Neal D. Barnard is an adjunct associate Professor of Medicine at George Washington University of Medicine and President of the Physicians Committee for Responsible Medicine, a nonprofit organization that promotes preventive medicine, conducts clinical research, and encourages tougher standards for ethics and effectiveness in research. He is the author of numerous books including _Foods That Fight Pain_, _Dr. Neal Barnard's Program for Reversing Diabetes_, _Breaking the Food Seduction_, _Turn Off the Fat Genes_, and, _Eat Right, Live Longer_.

Dr. T. Colin Campbell is a Jacob Gould Schurman Professor Emeritus of Nutritional Biochemistry at Cornell University. He has been a nutrition researcher for over 40 years and served as director of the China Study, the most comprehensive study of diet, lifestyle, and disease ever done with humans in the history of biomedical research. The New York Times described the project as the "Grand Prix of Epidemiology."

Brenda Davis is a registered dietitian and co-author of _Becoming Vegetarian_, and _Becoming Vegan_. Her other books include _Dairy-Free and Delicious, Defeating Diabetes_ and _The New Becoming Vegetarian_. She is a past chairperson of the Vegetarian Nutrition Dietetic Practice Group of the American Dietetic Association.

Reprinted with permission by Zel and Reuben Allen from the article entitled, _Calcium Basics_, from their website www.vegpradise.com, along with the following calcium source charts.

Calcium in Raw Nuts and Seeds (shelled)	
Nut/Seed (1 ounce)	**Calcium Milligrams**
Almonds (23)	70.0
Brazil nuts (6 to 8)	45.0
Cashews (18)	10.0
Chestnuts, Chinese boiled	3.0
Chestnut, European boiled	13.0
Chestnuts, Japanese roasted	10.0
Coconut meat, dried unsweetened	7.4
Hazelnuts/Filberts (21)	32.0
Flaxseeds (tablespoon ground)	18.0
Macadamias (10 to 12)	24.0
Peanuts, dry roasted	15.0
Pecans (19 halves)	20.0
Pine nuts	2.0
Pistachio (49)	30.0
Pumpkin seed (142)	12.0
Sesame seed, roasted	37.0
Sunflower seed, roasted	16.0
Walnut, black	17.0
Walnut, English (14 halves)	28.0
Watermelon seed, dried	15.0

Calcium in Beans
(dried, cooked)

Bean 1 cup	Calcium Milligrams
Adzuki Beans (Aduki)	64.0
Black Beans	46.0
Black-eyed Peas (Cowpeas)	39.0
Cranberry Beans	88.0
Fava Beans (Broadbeans)	61.0
Garbanzos (Chickpeas)	80.0
Great Northern Beans	120.0
Kidney Beans	50.0
Lentils	38.0
Lima Beans, large	32.0
Mung Beans	15.0
Navy Beans	126.0
Pink Beans	88.0
Pinto Beans	79.0
Soybeans	175.0
Split Peas	27.0

Calcium in Grains (cooked)	
Grain 1 cup	**Calcium Milligrams**
Amaranth	276.0
Barley, pearled	17.0
Buckwheat groats (kasha)	12.0
Bulgur Wheat	18.0
Hominy, canned	16.0
Millet, hulled	5.0
Oat bran	22.0
Rice, brown (long grain)	20.0
Rice, white	16.0
Rice, wild	5.0
Wheat, sprouted	30.0
Wheat bran, crude	42.0
Wheat germ. toasted	51.0

Calcium in Meat, Chicken, Fish Substitutes*

Product	Serving Size	Calcium Milligrams
Boca Burger Original Vegan	2.5 ounces	60
Dr. Praeger's Veggie Burgers	3 ounces	40
Health is Wealth Chicken-Free Patties	3 ounces	120
Lightlife Gimme Lean	2 ounces	40 to 60
Lightlife Ground Round	2 ounces	80
Lightlife Breakfast Links	2 links (2 ounces)	60
Soyrizo Chorizo	2 ounces	60
White Wave Tempeh	3 ounces	60
Yves Meatless Beef Burger	3 ounces	60
Yves Meatless Chicken Burgers	3 ounces	80
Yves Veggie Breakfast Patties	2 ounces	60
Yves Veggie Breakfast Links	3 ounces	80

*All items vegan

Calcium in Ready-to Eat Cereals		
Cereal	**Cup**	**Calcium Milligrams**
General Mills Basic 4	1	250.0
General Mills Cheerios	1	100.0
General Mills Fiber One	1	200.0
General Mills Total	3/4	258.0
General Mills Total Corn Flakes	1 1/3	1000.0
General Mills Total Raisin Bran	1	1000.0
General Mills Wheaties	1	20.0
Kellogg's All-Bran	1/2	121.0
Kellogg's Product 19	1	5.0
Kellogg's Raisin Bran	1	29.0
Kellogg's Rice Krispies	1	2.0
Kellogg's Special K	1	9.0
Post Grape Nuts	1/2	20.0
Post 100% Bran	1/3	22.0
Post Raisin Bran	1	30.0
Post Shredded Wheat	1 1/4	27.0
Quaker Cinnmon Life	1	138.0
Quaker Oat Bran	1 1/4	109.0
Quaker Oat Life Plain	3/4	112.0
Quaker 100% Natural Granola Oats & Honey	1/2	61.0

Calcium in Fresh Vegetables
(cooked)

Vegetable	Serving	Calcium Milligrams
Artichokes	medium	54.0
Asparagus	1/2 cup	21.0
Beans, Green	1 cup	55.0
Beet greens	1 cup	164.0
Beets, sliced	1 cup	28.0
Bok Choy (Chinese Cabbage)	1 cup	158.0
Broccoli, chopped	1/2 cup	31.0
Broccoli, Chinese	1 cup	88.0
Broccoli raab (Rapini)	1 bunch	516.0
Brussels Sprouts	1/2 cup	28.0
Cabbage, Green	1/2 cup	36.0
Cabbage, Red	1/2 cup	32.0
Cabbage, Savoy	1 cup	44.0
Carrots, sliced	1/2 cup	23.0
Cauliflower	1/2 cup	10.0
Celeriac	1 cup	40.0
Celery	1 cup diced	63.0
Chayote	1 cup	21.0
Collards	1 cup	266.0
Corn, Sweet	1 large ear	2.0
Dandelion Greens	1 cup	147.0
Eggplant	1 cup	6.0
Kale	1 cup	94.0
Kale, Scotch	1 cup	172.0
Kohlrabi,slices	1 cup	41.0
Leeks	1 medium	37.0
Okra, sliced	1/2 cup	62.0
Onions	1 cup	46.0
Parsnips	1/2 cup	29.0
Peas	1/2 cup	43.0

Peppers, green bell	1/2 cup	6.0
Potato medium, baked with skin	2 1/4" x 3 1/4"	26.0
Potato, boiled with skin	1/2 cup	4.0
Snow Peas	1 cup	94.0
Spinach	1 cup	245.0*
Squash, Acorn	1 cup cubed	90.0
Squash, Butternut	1 cup cubed	84.0
Squash, Crookneck	1 cup cubed	40.0
Squash, Hubbard	1 cup cubed	35.0
Squash, pattypan (summer scallop)	1 cup sliced	27.0
Squash, Spaghetti	1 cup	33.0
Squash, Winter	1 cup	29.0
Sweet Potato	1 medium with skin (2" x 5")	43.0
Swiss Chard	1 cup chopped	102*
Tomato, Stewed	1 cup	26.0
Turnip mashed	1 cup	26.0
Turnip greens	1 cup chopped	197.0
Zucchini	1 cup sliced	23.0

*Oxalates prevent the complete absorption of calcium.

Lettuce, romaine shredded

Calcium in Fresh Vegetables (raw)		
Vegetable	Serving	Calcium Milligrams
Artichoke	medium	56.0
Asparagus	1 cup	32.0
Beans, green	1 cup	41.0
Beans, kidney (Sprouted)	1 cup	31.0
Beans, mung (Sprouted)	1 cup	14.0
Beans, navy (Sprouted)	1 cup	16.0
Beets	1 cup	22.0
Broccoli	1/2 cup	21.0
Broccoli, Chinese	1 cup	88.0
Brussels Sprouts	1 cup	37.0
Cabbage, Chinese (Bok choy) shredded	1 cup	74.0
Cabbage, Chinese (Pe tsai) shredded	1 cup	59.0
Cabbage, green shredded	1 cup	28.0
Cabbage, red shredded	1 cup	32.0
Cabbage, savoy shredded	1 cup	24.0
Carrot, chopped	1 cup	42.0
Cauliflower	1 cup	22.0
Celeriac	1 cup	67.0
Celery, chopped	1 cup	40.0
Chayote, 1" pieces	1 cup	22.0
Collards, chopped	1 cup	52.0
Corn, Sweet	1 large ear	3.0
Dandelion Greens, chopped	1 cup	103.0
Fennel	1 medium bulb	115.0
Kale, chopped	1 cup	90.0
Kohlrabi	1 cup	32.0
Leeks	1 cup	53.0
Lettuce, butter shredded	1 cup	19.0
Lettuce, green leaf shredded	1 cup	13.0
Lettuce, iceberg shredded	1 cup	13.0
Lettuce, red leaf shredded	1 cup	9.0

1 cup	16.0	
Mustard Greens, chopped	1 cup	58.0
Okra	1 cup	81.0
Onions, chopped	1 cup	37.0
Parsnips, sliced	1 cup	48.0
Peas	1 cup	42.0
Peppers, bell, chopped	1 cup	15.0
Radish, red sliced	1 cup	29.0
Radish, White Icicle	1/2 cup	14.0
Snow Peas	1 cup	27.0
Spinach	1 cup	30.0*
Squash, acorn cubed	1 cup	46
Squash, butternut cubed	1 cup	67
Squash, crookneck cubed	1 cup	27
Squash, hubbard cubed	1 cup	16
Squash, spaghetti	1 cup	23.0
Sweet Potato, cubes	1 cup	40.0
Swiss Chard*	1 cup	18.0*
Tomato	3 inch	18.0
Turnip, cubes	1 cup	39.0
Turnip greens	1 cup	104.0
Zucchini, chopped	1 cup	19.0

*Oxalates prevent the complete absorption of calcium.

Calcium in Fruits (raw)		
Fruit	**Serving**	**Calcium Milligrams**
Apple	2 per pound	13.0
Apricot	1 medium	5.0
Avocado, California	1 medium	18.0
Avocado, Florida	1 mediium	30.0
Banana	9 inch	8.0
Blackberries	1 cup	42.0
Blueberries	1 cup	9.0
Boysenberries	1 cup frozen	36.0
Cantaloupe	1 cup cubed	17.6
Casaba Melon	1 cup cubed	14.0
Cherimoya (Custard Apple)	1 fruit	25.0
Cherries	1 cup	19.0
Cranberries	1 cup raw whole	8.0
Currants, Black	1 cup	62.0
Currants, Red/White	1 cup	37.0
Durian	1 cup chopped	15.0
Feijoa	1 med. trimmed	8.0
Fig	1 large (2.5") fig	22.0
Gooseberry	1 cup	38.0
Grape, Red or Green	1 cup	15.0
Grapefruit, Pink	1	15.0
Grapefruit, Red	1/2	27.0
Grapefruit. White	1/2	14.0
Guava	1 cup chopped	30.0
Guava, Strawberry	1 cup chopped	51.0
Honeydew	1 cup cubed	11.0
Jackfruit	1 cup siced	56.0
Kiwi	1 large	31.0
Kumquat	1 medium	12.0
Lemon	1 fruit 2 3/8 "	22.0

Lime	1 lime 2"	22.1
Loganberries	1 cup frozen	38.0
Loquat	1 medium	3.0
Mango	1 cup sliced	16.0
Mulberry	1 cup	54.6
Nectarine	1 fruit 2.5"	9.0
Orange, Florida	1 fruit 2 5/8"	61.0
Orange, navel	1 fruit 2 7/8"	48.0
Orange, valencia	1 fruit 2 5/8"	60.0
Papaya	1 cup cubed	34.0
Peach	1 medium 2 2/3"	9.0
Pear	1 pear medium	16.0
Persimmon	1 fruit 2.5"	7.0
Pineapple	1 cup diced	20.0
Plum	1 plum 2 1/8"	4.0
Pomegranate	1 fruit 3 3/8"	5.0
Prickly Pear	1 medium	58.0
Quince	1 medium	10.0
Raspberries	1 cup	31.0
Sapodilla	1 medium	36.0
Sapote (marmalade plum)	1 medium	88.0
Starfruit (carambola)	1 fruit 4.5"	4.0
Strawberries	1 cup whole	23.0
Tangerine (mandarin orange)	1 fruit 2.5"	33.0
Watermelon	1 cup diced	11.0

Calcium in Dried Fruits

Fruit	Serving	Calcium Milligrams
Apples	1/2 cup	6.0
Apricots	1/2 cup halves	36.0
Banana chips	1 1/2 ounces	8.0
Cranberries, dried sweetened	1/3 cup	4.0
Currants, zante	1/2 cup	62.0
Dates, deglet noor	1/2 cup pitted chopped	34.5
Dates, medjool	1 date	15.0
Figs	1/2 cup chopped	120.5
Peaches	1/2 cup halves	22.4
Pears	1/2 cup halves	22.5
Persimmons, Japanese	1 fruit	8.0
Prunes	1/2 cup pitted	37.5
Raisins, dark	1/2 cup	36.0
Raisins, golden	1/2 cup	43.5

Calcium in Nut/Seed Butters	
Nut/Seed (1 Tablespoon)	Calcium Milligrams
Almond	43.0
Cashew	7.0
Peanut	7.0
Sesame Tahini	64

Calcium in Milk Substitutes	
Beverage 1 cup	Calcium Milligrams
Soy milk, fortified	200.0 to 368.0
Soy milk, unfortified	93.0
Rice milk, Fortified	250 to 300
Almond, Fortified	200 to 300
Hazelnut, Fortified	300
Hempmilk	460

Calcium in Soy Products		
Product	**Serving Size**	**Calcium Milligrams**
Baked Tofu Medium to Extra Firm	3 ounces	100 to 150
Tofu with calcium Medium to Extra Firm	3 ounces	100 to 150
Tofu Soft or Silken	3 ounces	20 to 40
Tempeh	3 ounces	60
Textured Vegetable Protein TVP	1/4 cup	80
Soy Yogurt	8 ounces	150 to 300

Calcium in Miscellaneous Products		
Product	**Serving Size**	**Calcium Milligrams**
Blackstrap Molasses	1 tablespoon	172
Orange Juice, Fortified	8 ounce glass	300

Chapter 15

Where Do You Get Your Protein?

"If you don't eat meat, chicken, or fish, where do you get your protein?"

"You don't eat dairy products or eggs either? How can you live without protein?"

"You can't get enough protein on a vegan diet."

"My doctor told me I cannot stay healthy on a vegan diet."

"I tried a vegetarian diet but I got sick."

"I was on a vegetarian diet but I was so tired. I needed more protein."

Vegetarians and vegans have heard these statements over and over. Myths such as these simply will not go away without the solid facts to prove otherwise. I've attempted to reassure friends and family who shake their heads and click their tongues in utter amazement that I've survived so many years on a vegan diet and still haven't keeled over from lack of proper nutrition. My only doctor visits consist of a checkup every few years with accompanying lab tests that continue to affirm my excellent health. But simply telling people about it apparently isn't enough.

The hard fact that constantly comes to the foreground is that the focus on protein borders on obsession in the countries of the Western Hemisphere. One glance at restaurant menus and the plates that come to the table is proof that the centerpiece of the meal is a large serving of meat, chicken or fish, frequently smothered in creamy sauces or melted cheese. The portions served in one meal alone come close to fulfilling a day's worth of protein needs.

The meat and dairy industries spend billions of dollars to project their message right into your shopping cart through television commercials, magazine ads, and grocery store ads. These powerful industries even recognized it was important to teach young children "good nutrition" at a very early age. Since the end of World War II they spread their protein message to our nation's youth by providing schools across the United States with colorful charts of the "important food groups" that emphasize meat, dairy products, and eggs. For the decades following World War II, one simply could not ignore the emphasis on protein.

Could we fail to ignore the large billboards flaunting larger-than-life-size images of cheese, eggs, and milk? And who can forget the successful ad campaigns for "Where's the beef" and "Milk does a body good?" The protein message comes at us from all directions, even at bus stops.

Please don't misunderstand, I fully recognize that protein is a necessity to a healthy body, and that it is important to replenish our store of protein every day. Because the body doesn't store protein as it does other nutrients, we are aware it must be replaced each day as a source of nourishment for building and repairing new cells, hormones, antibiotics, enzymes, and muscle tissue. But how much protein do we really need?

Recently, studies on nitrogen balance provided more accurate ways to measure the body's protein requirements. Joel Fuhrman, M.D. in his book **Eat to Live,** writes "… an easy way to calculate your own daily protein requirement according to the U.S. RDA is to multiply 0.36 g by your body weight (If you have a problem with grams keep in mind that 1 g equals 0.035 ounces). That translates to about 44 g for a 120 pound woman and 54 g for a 150 pound male, or 1-1/2 and 2 ounces respectively."

Brenda Davis, R. D. and Vesanto Melina, M.S., R.D., in their book, **Becoming Vegan**, consider 0.9 g per kilogram of body weight to be more ideal for vegans eating whole plant foods such as legumes, whole grains, and vegetables. Multiplying 0.45 g or 0.035 ounces by your body weight in pounds will give you the approximate protein needs for your body. These figures are a little higher than the actual RDA requirements but were considered necessary as a safety factor to account for reduced digestibility of whole plant foods versus more refined foods such as tofu and meat substitutes. With the slightly higher figure, a 120-pound person would need 54 g of protein daily, or 2 ounces of protein, and a 150-pound person needs 67.5 g or roughly 2-1/4 ounces of protein daily.

The newest RDA has looked at all the places where additional protein is needed in pregnancy (fetus, placenta, amniotic fluid, uterus, breasts, blood, etc.) and has recommended that protein intake and pregnancy should be 25 g or roughly 1 ounce more of protein than the RDA for non-pregnant women. The same recommendation is made for lactation to account for the protein content of milk.

During pregnancy and breast-feeding, protein needs can easily be met by adding a little extra of the foods higher in protein, such as enriched soy milk, beans, tofu, tempeh, nuts and nut butters, in addition to a wide variety of fruits and vegetables.

While the focus on protein is important, the green leafy vegetables such as collards, kale, mustard greens, turnip greens, and spinach are also necessary for their high content of folate to prevent neural tube defects such as spina bifida.

Patients recuperating from surgery or serious bodily injuries, such as burns, require extra protein to help rebuild tissue. Their protein intake should be at a level of about 20% of their calorie intake.

If you're an athlete or one who works at serious bodybuilding, one or more of your trainers may have suggested using protein powders or amino acid powders on a regular basis. Sports nutrition has focused heavily on protein.

In relating the position of the newest RDA information, professional athletes may need more protein than those who are not in serious training, but how much more and even whether or not their protein needs are higher is a matter of differing opinion. I think the research supports slightly higher protein needs for athletes, but not everyone goes along with this.

A diet that consists of 12% to 15% protein is considered ideal for both strength and endurance for athletes who follow a vegan diet. For vegan athletes who want to keep their body weight low, 15% to 20% of calories should be protein. About 10% to 12% of calories as protein may be all that is required of those on very high calorie diets, such as Ironman athletes.

Dr. Ruth Heidrich, a vegan Ironman athlete, expresses the protein needs of athletes very simply. She says,"With greater calorie burning comes greater calorie consumption with its automatic increase in the absolute amount of protein." For people who want to build more muscle, Dr. Heidrich discourages the use of protein supplements and stresses that, "If you want to develop a muscle, you have to overload it by putting more stress on it than it can handle. This is the ONLY way a muscle would get bigger and stronger."

If a person is eating a broad selection of plant-based foods and consuming adequate calories, it is unlikely he or she will be protein deficient. Physicians in the United States rarely encounter patients who are deficient in protein. Deficiency is uncommon and is seen mostly in countries where serious shortages of food exist, and malnutrition is prevalent.

More common are the problems resulting from eating too much protein. In contrast to the U.S. RDA calculations, the average person in America consumes foods containing 100 to 120 g of protein daily or 352 to 420 ounces, mostly from animal products. Americans are also noted for their sedentary lifestyles. Excess protein, especially of animal nature, puts a great deal of stress on the kidneys. Some people, unaware that their kidneys are not operating optimally, could suffer premature aging of this important organ. A diet too high in protein could cause deterioration of the nephrons, which are the kidney's filtering system. That same diet places people at risk for developing kidney stones.

Other health conditions that may result from the overabundance of protein include excessive calcium leaching from the bones and causing osteoporosis, acid reflux, obesity, plaque build-up in the arteries, high blood pressure, pain from arthritis, high cholesterol, bad breath from sulfur-containing amino acids (not to be confused with Organic Sulfur Crystals), and increased risk of cancer, especially colon cancer.

The following charts, using figures from the USDA Nutrient Database, list the protein content of the plant-based foods that comprise the vegetarian and vegan diets. People are often surprised to learn that all plant foods contain protein. In fact, it is protein that gives all plants their structure. Whether plants grow upright or sprawl on a vine, protein is a basic component of their cell structure.

This article was re-printed with permission by Zel and Reuben Allen of www.vegparadise.com along with the following protein source charts.

Protein in Raw Nuts and Seeds (shelled)

Nut/Seed (1/4 cup)	Protein Grams
Almond	7
Brazil nut	5
Cashew	4
Chestnut	1
Coconut (shredded)	2
Filbert/Hazelnut	5
Flax seed	5
Macadamia	2
Peanut	8
Pecan	2
Pine nut	4
Pistachio	6
Pumpkin seed	7
Sesame seed	7
Soynut	10
Sunflower seed	8
Walnut	5

Protein in Beans (cooked)

Bean 1 cup	Protein Grams
Adzuki (Aduki)	17
Anasazi	15
Black Beans	15
Black-eyed Peas	14
Cannellini (White Beans)	17
Cranberry Bean	17
Fava Beans	13
Garbanzos (Chick Peas)	15
Great Northern Beans	15
Green Peas, whole	9
Kidney Beans	15
Lentils	18
Lima Beans	15
Mung Beans	14
Navy Beans	16
Pink Beans	15
Pinto Beans	14
Soybeans	29
Split Peas	16

Protein in Grains (cooked)

Grain 1 cup	Protein Grams
Amaranth	7
Barley, pearled	4 to 5
Barley, flakes	4
Buckwheat groats	5 to 6
Cornmeal (fine grind)	3
Cornmeal (polenta, coarse)	3
Millet, hulled	8.4
Oat Groats	6
Oat, bran	7
Quinoa	5
Rice, brown	3 to 5
Rice, white	4
Rice, wild	7
Rye, berries	7
Rye, flakes	6
Spelt, berries	5
Teff	6
Triticale	25
Wheat, whole berries	6 to 9
Couscous, whole wheat	6
Wheat, bulgur	5 to 6

Protein in Meat, Chicken, Fish Substitutes*

Product	Serving Size	Protein Grams
Boca Burger Original Vegan	2.5 oz	13
GardenVegan Veggie Patties	2.5 oz	9
Health is Wealth Chicken-Free Patties	3 oz.	14
Health is Wealth Yummie Burger	2.5 oz.	12
Lightlife Gimme Lean	2oz.	8
Lightlife Smart Cutlets Seasoned Chicken	3 oz.	26
Lightlife Smart Deli Combos	2.7 oz.	17
Lightlife Smart Dogs	1.5 oz.	9
Mon Cuisine Breaded Chicken Patties	3 oz.	7
Morningstar Farms Original Grillers	2.3 oz	15
Nate's Meatless Meatballs (3)	1.5 oz	10
Natural Touch Vegan Burger	2.7 oz	11
Natural Touch Veggie Medley	2.3 oz	11
SoyBoy Vegan Okara Burger	3 oz.	13
SoyBoy Vegetarian Franks	1.5 oz.	11
Starlite Cuisine Soy Taquitos	2 oz.	7
White Wave Seitan	3 oz.	31
Whole Foods 365 Meat Free Vegan Burger	2.5 oz.	13
Yves Canadian Veggie Bacon (3 slices)	2 oz.	17
Yves Veggie Burger	3 oz.	16
Yves Veggie Chick'n Burgers	3 oz.	17
Yves Veggie Dogs	1.6 oz.	11

*All items vegan

Protein in Hot Cereals (cooked)

Cereal	Cup	Protein Grams
Arrowhead Mills Corn Grits	1/4	3
Arrowhead Mills 7 Grain	1/4	4
Bob's 8 Grain	1/4	4
Bob's 10 Grain	1/4	6
Bob's Kamut	1/4	5
Bob's Triticale	1/4	4
Bob's Whole Grain Cracked Wheat	1/4	5
Cream of Rye	1/3	5
Kashi	1/2	6
Mother's Multigrain	1/2	5
Quaker Old Fashioned Oats	1/2	5
Quinoa Flakes	1/3	3
Roman Meal Hot Cereal	1/3	5
Wheatena	1/3	5

Protein in Fresh Vegetables (cooked)

Vegetable	Serving	Protein Grams
Artichoke	medium	4
Asparagus	5 spears	2
Beans, string	1 cup	2
Beets	1/2 cup	1
Broccoli	1/2 cup	2
Brussels Sprouts	1/2 cup	2
Cabbage	1/2 cup	1
Carrot	1/2 cup	1
Cauliflower	1/2 cup	1
Celeriac	1 cup	1
Celery	1 cup	1
Chard, Swiss	1 cup	3
Chayote	1 cup	1
Chives	1 tablespoon	0.10
Collards	1 cup	4
Corn, Sweet	1 large cob	5
Cucumber	1 cup	1
Eggplant	1 cup	1
Fennel	1 medium bulb	3
Jerusalem Artichoke	1 cup	3
Kale	1 cup	2.5
Kohlrabi	1 cup	3
Leeks	1 cup	1
Lettuce	1 cup	1
Okra	1/2 cup	1
Onion	1/2 cup	1
Parsnip	1/2 cup	1
Peas	1/2 cup	4
Peppers, bell	1/2 cup	1

Potato, baked with skin	2 1/3 x 4 3/4"	5
Potato, boiled with skin	1/2 cup	1
Radish	1 cup	1
Rhubarb	1 cup	1
Rutabaga	1 cup	2
Spinach	1 cup	1
Squash, Summer	1 cup	2
Squash, Winter	1 cup	2
Sweet Potato	1 cup	3
Tomato	1 medium	1
Turnip	1 cup	1

Protein in Fruits (raw)

Fruit	Serving	Protein Grams
Apple	2 per lb.	0
Apricot	med.	0
Avocado	med.	4
Banana	1	1 to 2
Blackberry	cup	2
Blueberry	cup	1
Boysenberry	cup	1
Cantaloupe	cup	1
Casaba Melon	cup	2
Cherimoya	1	7
Cherry	cup	1
Cranberry	cup	0
Currant	cup	2
Date(pitted)	1/4 cup	1
Durian	1 cup	4
Feijoa	med.	1
Fig	1	0
Gooseberry	cup	1
Grape	cup	1
Grapefruit	1/2	1
Guava	med.	1
Honeydew	cup	1
Jackfruit	cup	2
Jujube, dried	1 oz.	1
Kiwi	large	1
Kumquat	med.	0
Lemon	1	1
Lime	1	0
Loganberry	cup	1.4

Loquat	1	0
Mango	1	1
Mulberry	cup	2
Nectarine	1	1
Orange	1	1
Papaya	cup	1
Passionfruit	1	0
Peach	1	1
Pear	1	1
Persimmon	1	0
Pineapple	cup	1
Plum	1	1
Pomegranate	1	1.5
Pomelo	1/2	2.3
Prickly Pear	med.	1
Quince	med.	.4
Raspberry	cup	1
Rhubarb	cup	1
Sapote	med.	5
Star Fruit	cup	1
Strawberry	cup	1
Tangerine	med.	1
Watermelon	cup	1

Protein in Nut Butters

Nut/Seed (2 Tablespoons)	Protein Grams
Almond	5 to 8
Cashew	4 to 5
Peanut	7 to 9
Sesame Tahini	6
Soy Nut	6 to 7

Protein in Milk Substitutes

Beverage 1 cup	Protein Grams
Soy Regular	6 to 9
Soy Low/Nonfat	4
Rice	1
Rice and Soy	7
Almond	1 to 2
Oat	4
Multigrain	5

Protein in Soy Products

Product	Serving Size	Protein Grams
Tofu Medium to Extra Firm	3 oz.	7 to 12
Tofu Soft or Silken	3 oz.	4 to 6
Tempeh	4 oz.	12 to 20
Textured Vegetable Protein TVP	1/4 cup	10 to 12

Chapter 16

Crossing The Bridge

M any times, when people try to make the switch to vegetarianism they are basically clueless. When I was faced with that transition, the person that introduced me to vegetarianism bailed and I was in a quandary. Yet, I survived and survived very nicely.

This chapter, which was originally entitled "The Road to Vegetaria," appeared on the Vegetarians in Paradise website. Its purpose was to enlighten people about the transitional alternatives available to them as a vegetarian. So, let's give it a shot.

MEAT ALTERNATIVES

Instead Of Meat:

Explore the world of TOFU. Made from soybeans, TOFU is very high in protein; the firmer it is, the higher the protein content and the less water it contains. When processed with calcium sulfate, TOFU is a good source of calcium. TOFU is one of the most versatile foods available for vegetarians.

TOFU can be prepared in any of the following ways: marinated, sautéed, steamed, braised, roasted, baked, broiled, stir-fried, deep fried, mashed, blended, or puréed in a food processor.

There are other meat alternatives in the deli case of your natural foods store. SEITAN, made from wheat gluten, is high in protein and can lend a meat-like texture to many dishes. SEITAN can be sliced, ground, chopped, or diced and will readily absorb definitive seasonings when cooked in a stir-fry, casserole, or in a well seasoned sauce.

TEMPEH is a formatted soybean cake that improves with marinating and makes a hearty high-protein substitute for meat. It can be baked, broiled, chopped, shredded, sautéed, stir fried, and braised. TEMPEH is an excellent addition to casseroles, pastas, stir-fries, salads, wraps, soups, and ethnic dishes like tacos, burritos, chili, sushi, and curries. Try marinating chopped TEMPEH and adding it to a pita sandwich along with chopped or shredded veggies and your favorite dressing.

NUTS AND SEEDS are excellent meat replacements, high in protein, fiber, essential fatty acids, and vitamin E. Nuts are an outstanding source of minerals, including calcium, iron, zinc, and copper. A serving of 2 ounces of nuts several times a week lowers the risk for heart attack, diabetes, and gallstones, and lowers total and LDL cholesterol. Make sure the NUTS AND SEEDS you purchase are raw, not roasted in oil or assaulted. To keep them fresh for several weeks, refrigerate them to prevent rancidity.

Instead of Beef Broth:

Choose low-sodium canned or packaged vegetable broth or create your own flavorful broth with a base of vegetables and water. To season the broth, add a small amount of TAMARI, BRAGG'S LIQUID AMINOS, or low-sodium SOY SAUCE, a clove of garlic, perhaps a squeeze of fresh lemon juice, and season with your favorite herbs, salt, and pepper. Keep in mind, when dealing with soy, because so much of it is genetically modified, you should try to buy strictly organic.

To turn the broth into GRAVY, thicken by combining equal parts of cornstarch or arrowroot and water (about 2 tablespoons each for 2 cups broth) and stir into a smooth, runny paste. Add the paste to gently simmering broth a little at a time, stirring constantly for about one minute, or until thickened to the desired consistency.

VEGETABLE BOUILLON CUBES in imitation beef flavor are easily dissolved in boiling water to create a quick beef flavored broth. Plant based POWDERED BEEF FLAVORING is also a quick method for making beef broth alternatives. Both are available in natural foods stores. Look for low-sodium options.

Instead Of Hamburgers:

Awaken to the joy of VEGGIE BURGERS. They won't really fool you into believing they are beef but they sure are impressive substitutes. Enjoy your VEGGIE BURGER on a whole-grain hamburger bun or tucked into a pita with the usual fixings like lettuce, tomato, onion, pickles, ketchup, and mustard, and top it off with a slice of vegan cheese, if desired. Trust me, you won't miss the beef!

Some of the better brands to look for, in my opinion, are Sunshine and Maui Taro Burgers. There are many more however, including Amy's, Boca, and Gardenburger. But, I stopped eating those long ago because they use euphemistic MSG as flavoring.

Instead Of Hot Dogs:

Several food manufacturers produce VEGETARIAN HOT DOGS made from soy protein. Many are fat-free. You'll have to check out the different brands for yourself to find the one you like best. Then tucked into a whole-grain hot dog bun, cover it with mustard, relish, and sauerkraut, and you will never look back.

Instead Of Turkey:

There's a product out there called TOFURKY. It looks like Turkey, it's shaped like Turkey, but it's not turkey. For Thanksgiving, it makes a great alternative.

CHICKEN ALTERNATIVES

Instead Of Chicken:

Explore the multitude of frozen chicken substitutes made from soy protein and wheat gluten. Tastes and textures are very close to the real thing, and you will benefit from a reduced intake of saturated fat and eliminate the cholesterol altogether.

LEGUMES include a huge variety of beans, lentils, split green or yellow peas, and are delicious high-protein alternatives to animal products. Begin by choosing one night a week to prepare a dish that features legumes as the centerpiece of your meal. Build a special dish by combining your beans with vegetables and your favorite seasonings or sauces and come away from the table feeling comfortably full rather than heavy and overstuffed. As you become more accustomed to plant-based foods, you may enjoy two or three nights or even whole days in being completely vegetarian.

The varieties of BEANS are numerous and each one has a uniquely different taste and texture. Explore black beans, garbanzo beans, pinto beans, lima beans, fava beans, kidney beans, black-eyed peas, northern beans, navy beans, yellow and green split peas, and lentils of many colors and sizes.

Instead Of Chicken Broth:

Purchase a vegetarian imitation chicken broth, available in powdered form that can be dissolved in water. Alternatively, create your own beginning with 2 or 3 cups of water. Add a bit of soy sauce or Bragg's amino liquid, some nutritional yeast, a touch of lemon juice, and a bit of salt and pepper. For a creamy style broth, add some organic soymilk or rice milk.

To turn the broth into gravy, stir together equal parts of cornstarch or arrowroot and water (about 2 tablespoons each for 2 cups of liquid) into a smooth runny paste. Add the paste a little at a time to gently simmering broth, stirring constantly for about one minute or until thickened. Simmer gently for one minute longer.

FISH ALTERNATIVES

Instead Of Fish:

Many Asian markets will have fish flavored soy protein in the freezer section. They are innovatively created to look like the real thing. Some varieties come in fish-steak slabs with nori seaweed wrapped around the outer edge to resemble the skin of a fish. However, one thing that's important to remember is to read the ingredient labels very carefully. Some of the imitation fish may contain whey or casein - milk protein used as binders.

DAIRY ALTERNATIVES

Instead Of Butter:

Enjoy the richness of spreading one fourth of a ripe avocado on your bread or toast. Historically, avocados were known as midshipmen's butter and were used in England's Royal Navy in the 1800s. Avocados are creamy, delicious, and offer naturally beneficial fats.

NUT BUTTERS are other bread spread alternatives. These nut butters include peanut, almond, macadamia, or cashew. Be sure to purchase brands that contain only roasted nuts. Be sure to avoid those nut butters with unnecessary ingredients like sugar, salt, and partially hydrogenated oils a.k.a. trans-fats. Nut butters are delicious, healthful and contain ample protein.

SEED BUTTERS, made from roasted sesame seeds or sunflower seeds are another alternative. TAHINI, which is sesame seed paste, is a good source of calcium and tastes great on whole-grain pita bread or crackers. If the tahini seems a little bland, try a light sprinkle of salt or herbs such as cumin, like the ancient Romans did.

Other spreads to try including TOFU SPREADS, HUMMUS, a tasty Middle Eastern dish made from garbanzo beans, and FRUIT BUTTERS, which are naturally sweet and delicious.

When you sauté vegetables, be sure to replace the unhealthy fats like butter with water, vegetable broth, or olive oil. When sautéing with olive oil do not use extra-virgin olive oil as it has a low heat tolerance. Use extra-virgin olive oil on raw foods.

Instead Of Milk, Cream, Or Cheese

On your cereal, switch to organic soymilk, rice milk, oat milk or hemp milk. If you use almond milk, be careful that the almonds do not come from California as all California almonds are irradiated. When you use these various milk alternatives, be sure to read labels, as some of these are high in sugar.

To create a cream sauce with a delicate cheese flavor, add a tablespoon or two of nutritional yeast flakes, which are high in vitamin B12, to any of the above-mentioned alternatives.

Instead of cream cheese, sour cream, or regular high-fat cheese, there is a wide variety of low fat, vegan substitutes found in the coolers of your local health food store.

EGG ALTERNATIVES

Instead Of Egg Salad:

You can purchase MOCK EGG SALAD made from tofu or prepare your own version from an easy basic recipe with regular or firm tofu. Here's a basic recipe to get you started:

Start with a package of extra firm tofu. Open it and drain all the liquid. Next you need a frying pan to which you will add some olive oil. Slice up some onions and mushrooms and cut red and green bell peppers into small pieces. Throw it all in the frying pan. After it is cooked for a bit take the tofu and mash it in your hands, dropping it into the frying pan. You can also finally cut a potato and add that as well. As far as spices go, I like to use garlic powder, a little bit of Bragg's Aminos, some turmeric, and a bit of hot sauce. Then continue to fry up the whole batch.

Instead of using eggs for baking, there's a product out there called: ENER-G-EGG REPLACER. It works just as well as eggs and doesn't give you any cholesterol as it is made from potato starch, tapioca flour, and a few other things that are not at all harmful. You can find that in your natural foods store. You use 1 teaspoon of ENER-G to 2 tablespoons of water for each egg.

MAYONNAISE ALTERNATIVE

Instead Of Mayonnaise:

There is a product out there called FOLLOW YOUR HEART VEGENAISE. It is a totally vegan alternative that tastes just like the real thing. Even though this mayonnaise alternative does not contain cholesterol it is a bit high in fat. Recently they came out with a variety that is lower in fat. It contains flax seed oil. It's a great product.

WHOLE GRAIN ALTERNATIVES

By this time most people know the difference between white breads and whole grain breads. But just to be safe, look for words like "whole grain wheat flour" and "100% whole wheat flour," rather than "enriched wheat flour." In this case, "White ain't right!" Also, look for multigrain breads for their wholesome richness and flavor as well as benefits from the extra nutrition. When you read the labels choose the breads that have at least 3 g of fiber per slice, preferably 4 or 5. The higher the fiber content of the food, the better it is for your digestive tract.

You can also experiment with many whole-grain pastas that undoubtedly will be new to you. Pastas made from whole wheat, quinoa, spelt, rice, buckwheat, and barley, will offer a treat to your taste buds.

Believe it or not, most whole-grain hot cereals take no more than five minutes to prepare. Old-fashioned oatmeal makes a great start to the day, as its soluble fiber helps to lower cholesterol naturally. If you want to take a "walk on the wild side" when you prepare your oatmeal, try this: After you put the oats in the saucepan add some vanilla rice milk. Then, put in some sliced bananas, strawberries, and blueberries. Cook it that way and your taste buds will explode.

Instead of white rice, try brown rice, quinoa, buckwheat, or millet. They might take a bit longer to cook, but there is no comparison to the nutrition you will receive.

SUGAR ALTERNATIVES

Instead Of Refined White Sugar:

EVAPORATED CANE JUICE is sugar cane that has had the water removed or evaporated. This sugar has not gone through the last step in the typical refining process of granulated sugar, a step which involves clarifying the sugar over charred animal bones to make it white. While the evaporated cane juice may have an off-white color, it is totally vegan and it has the same level of sweetness as granulated sugar. Use it the same way.

STEVIA, although the Fraud and Drug Administration prohibits its labeling as a sweetener, is one of the best natural sweeteners on the planet. Stevia is a natural herb.

Then of course there are always others that you probably heard of like SUCANAT, made from whole cane juice, containing 100% of the natural molasses. MAPLE SYRUP, the natural sap from maple trees, is an excellent sweetener. This is not to be confused with "Log Cabin" or any of that other sugar-loaded garbage. If you're reading labels and you see BARLEY MALT, or BROWN RICE SYRUP, or DATE SUGAR, don't worry, it's safe.

INSTEAD OF ICE CREAM:

My favorite: SOY DELICIOUS NON-DAIRY ICE CREAM. With flavors like Mocha Fudge, Chocolate Obsession, Cherry Nirvana, Chocolate Velvet, Pomegranate Chip, Mint Chocolate Chip, and more, how can you go wrong? Bear in mind that a quart of Soy Delicious contains 32 teaspoons of sugar.

References: this article, originally entitled, 'The Road To Vegetaria' was reprinted with permission, and minor changes, from Zel and Ruben Allen of www. vegetariansinparadise.com

Chapter 17

"Fat, Fat, The Water Rat"

I f you are walking around with excess baggage around your waist and you can't get rid of it, there are 11 things that you might want to try.

1. You need to believe that the only thing that matters is the composition of the foods on your plate. Do not focus on anything else. Don't think about how much you eat. Don't think about exercise. It doesn't matter if you're a nice person, or if you go to church, or if a few classmates picked on you in high school. It's all in the food! All you have to do is permanently change your life. I sincerely mean this: to lose weight and regain your lost health, is to change the make-up of the meal that you put into your mouth.

2. You can learn the truth about permanent weight loss by simply opening your eyes. Look around the world. Who are the millions of people who looked trim, healthy and young, and have the physical shape that you want? Did you pick Japanese, Thai, Peruvians, or rural Mexicans? Did you also notice that although these people follow diets based on starches such as rice, beans, potatoes, and corn, they eat very little meat, dairy, and processed foods? They also avoid the diseases that are common to us. Change your meals to these comfort foods and solve your health and weight

problems. Make this simple observation and you will never be fooled by fad diets again.

3. The more you eat, the thinner and healthier you will become. You have tried low-calorie diets in the past. Most of these kinds of diets are based on restricting how much you eat. Do you remember the agonizing pains from hunger? How could you expect your willpower to win out? Each successive time you tried portion-controlled, calorie- restricted diets, you did worse than with previous attempts. The pain of hunger is a powerful teacher.

4. Rather than semi-starvation, during your most desperate times you ate all you could stomach of meat, cheese, and eggs. Does the Atkins Diet come to mind? You became ill with ketosis, lost your appetite and some weight. Being sick is unpleasant, so you had to cease this foolishness and you regained your lost weight. Now you worry about the possible long-term consequences of eating all that fat and cholesterol: cancer, heart disease, arthritis, hemorrhoids, etc.

5. If you have tried to follow a plant-based diet in the past and got off track, don't be discouraged. Pleasure is also a powerful teacher, like hunger. It is likely you remember this experience as a time when you felt your best, you lost weight effortlessly, and you were never hungry. Your body was feeling good and your future was promising. Now is the time to give a diet based on plants another chance -- and you would do better than you did the last time -- you'll follow this enlightened path more faithfully, and you will become stronger, trimmer, and more attractive as the months and years pass. To accelerate your weight loss, increase the quantity of green and yellow vegetables in your diet. But don't overdo the low-calorie cauliflower and pea pods. Starch must remain your source of clean, appetite-satisfying calories. Focus on whole grains, not refined flours, like those found in bagels and pretzels, white breads and white pastas.

6. Your goal should be to find a few meals that you really enjoy and are willing to fix over and over again. Dr. McDougall's website has published more than 2500 recipes. There is an endless supply of vegetarian cookbooks out there as well. Your goal is to find one dish you like for breakfast, one for lunch, and two or three for dinner. When someone asks: " What's for

dinner?" You say, "bean burritos, minestrone soup and whole grain bread, black bean chili, or pasta and marinara sauce." Think starch-centered meals.

7. The fat you eat is the fat you wear. You can expect that the fats from animal foods, such as meat, poultry, fish, milk and cheese, as well as, those found in large amounts in some plant foods, such as nuts, seeds, avocados and olives, will be effortlessly moved into and stored in your body fat. The most harmful sources of fat are concentrated animal forms, such as lard and butter, and those extracted from plants, such as olive, corn, safflower, and flaxseed oils. When mixed into soups, stews, and bakery products they seem to disappear, only to reappear around your waistline.

8. Under usual living situations, carbohydrates do not turn into body fat. Rather than being stored, excess carbohydrate calories are burned off as body heat, eliminated through the lungs and skin. Only by consuming very large amounts of refined flours and simple sugars will the body resort to converting carbohydrate into fat. Fructose, often present as high fructose corn syrup in fountain sodas and candies, is an exception in that this one form of simple carbohydrate is easily converted into body fat. Otherwise, think: "Carbohydrates found in rice, potatoes, broccoli and bananas will keep me fit and healthy, just like they do for people living in Asia and Peru."

9. Alcohol does not turn into fat. Friends who brag about their "beer belly" are mistaken. This is really "a pizza, cheese and potato chip fat belly." Excess alcohol calories are burned off as heat, not stored. Serious alcoholics are underweight. However, moderate drinking contributes to being overweight by providing readily usable, alcohol derived calories -- the body burns alcohol and leaves fat stored in your buttocks. Plus, alcohol reduces self-control causing you to be unable "to eat just one" of anything.

10. Exercise helps, but it cannot compensate for oil and sugar-filled foods. First manage every morsel that passes your lips, and then start burning a few more calories with exercise. Find something you love to do so that this valuable time is eagerly anticipated. When I play basketball, softball, racquetball, bodysurf or do martial arts, I call these activities pure pleasure - not exercise. Is there something you love doing? Tennis? Walking? Bicycling? Hiking? Just do it!

11. Eating out is a major downfall for most people. Do not make restaurants your chief cook. Even though you ask the waiter for "no-added-oil," you will more often than not be served a meal glistening with grease. If you do have to eat out, keep it simple, like baked potatoes, sweet potatoes, beans and brown rice. Or take one fine-dining establishment and challenge the chef to make you an oil-free creation of unrefined starches, vegetables, and fruits.

Follow these simple points and as you pass somebody, you will never again hear the song: "I feel the earth move under my feet."

References: this article was reprinted with permission and minor modification by Dr. John Mc Dougall from his website, www.drmcdougall.com. The original title of this article was:

' If I Could Be Your Doctor, I would Love To tell You How: To Lose Excess Weight Effortlessly, Painlessly, and Permanently'

Chapter 18

Class Is In Session

First, let's define the many categories that encompass the term "vegetarian." Often we hear people say that they no longer eat red meat, just chicken and fish, so they consider themselves vegetarians. These are not vegetarians, but we hope that some day their diet will evolve into becoming vegetarian. True vegetarians follow a diet that avoids animal flesh and emphasizes plant-based foods that consist of whole grains, legumes, fruits, vegetables, nuts and seeds.

LACTO-OVO VEGETARIAN: Eats no meat, poultry, or fish, but includes dairy products and eggs in the diet, along with plant-based foods.

LACTO VEGETARIAN: Excludes all animal products except dairy products. Includes all plant-based foods in the diet.

OVO VEGETARIAN: Excludes all animal products except eggs. Includes all plant-based foods in the diet.

VEGAN OR PURE VEGETARIAN: Vegan is pronounced "vee gun." Some people distinguish between vegan and pure vegetarian, considering the pure vegetarian one who eats no animal flesh, no dairy products, no eggs, and follows a strict plant-based diet for dietary reasons only. While vegans follow a diet consisting of plant-based foods only, they are further committed to a philosophy that does not put them at risk of being re-born in an animal body and not supporting the ecology of the planet.

As a result, many vegans also do not eat honey because many bees are killed in the process of forced procreation to maintain the beehive and the continued production of honey.

They do not eat refined cane sugar because it is clarified over animal bones in the final steps of the process that makes the sugar white. Instead, vegans choose unrefined sweeteners such as evaporated cane juice, maple sugar, maple syrup, date sugar, Sucanat, and agave nectar. Vegans also avoid gelatin, which is made from the bones, skin, and connective tissue of animals.

Because vegans consider the ecology of the planet a priority along with concern for animal rights, many shun the use of leather, wool, silk, goose down, and any foods or goods that have been processed using animal products. Their concern is that the planet's future resources have been harmed and animals have suffered in order for those products to come to market.

FRUITARIAN: The fruitarian has a simpler diet consisting only of seed-bearing fruits that include whole fresh fruits and some foods from the vine that are technically considered fruits, but have been used as vegetables. These vegetable/fruits comprise cucumbers, tomatoes, squashes, peppers and olives. Avocados, technically a tree fruit eaten as a vegetable, are also embraced. Fruitarians may also include coconuts, nuts and seeds, and some greens that they carefully harvest in a manner that allows the plant to continue producing leaves.

LIVING FOODS DIET: Those who follow the living foods diet call themselves, "live fooders" or "live foodists" and need a broad variety of fresh fruits, vegetables, soaked nuts and seeds, soaked and sprouted grains and legumes, and sea vegetables. They also include cultured foods such as live vegetable krauts, fermented nut and seed cheeses, and other cultured foods that contain friendly bacteria. Green drinks and soups, along with wheatgrass juice are encouraged, while stimulating and salty foods may be consumed sparingly. Food combining is important to maintain good digestion and a vigorous constitution. In addition, "live fooders" will warm some other foods in a dehydrator with a temperature regulator. In order to preserve the valuable enzymes that raw foods contain, some foods may be warmed to temperatures no higher than 105°, while others will tolerate a little higher heat, up to 115°.

NATURAL HYGIENE DIET: Those who follow the natural hygiene regimen consume a diet of whole, organically grown fresh fruits, vegetables, nuts and seeds in their raw, natural state, often eating only one food at a meal until satiated. They place a strong focus on proper food combining for optimal digestion and employ occasional water fasts. Natural fats such as avocados, nuts and seeds, are eaten in small quantities, while extracted vegetable oils are discouraged. Certain strong tasting foods are eschewed, such as: garlic, onions, sea vegetables, salt, fermented foods, and super green foods such as bluegreen algae. Other principles important to their lifestyle include fresh pure air, pure water, moderate sunshine, regular exercise, adequate sleep, and fasting when ill.

RAW FOODIST: included in their regimen are all fresh fruits, vegetables, nuts and seeds (raw as well as soaked and sprouted), and soaked and sprouted grains and legumes. Many enjoy low-temperature dehydrated crackers, cereals, sprouted raw breads, and fresh fruit and nut-based desserts. Those who follow the raw food diet are more flexible and inclusive of flavor-enhanced foods such as marinated fruits and vegetables. Surprisingly elegant gourmet foods have emerged from the raw food kitchen, yet many prefer simpler foods that require little preparation. Further, the "raw foodist" never cooks or warms the food on a stove, but eats them only in their natural, raw state in order to preserve their valuable enzymes.

The plant-based diet, at first thought, may seem rather limiting. Surprisingly though, this regimen offers much more variety than most people realize. There are many new products on the market that make the transition from a meat-based diet an enjoyable change. Change, however, can be challenging. The question that many face is whether to make this transition a gradual one or to plunge in dramatically? Generally, a gradual transition is more likely to help one stay on the vegetarian path.

Instead of planning your meal around meat, chicken, or fish as the centerpiece, think of whole grains or legumes as the centerpiece. Enhance the grains or legumes with your favorite seasonings, vegetables, nuts or seeds. Take a little extra time to make it special. Surround your special dish with steamed vegetables. Include a salad or two every day, made with dark leafy greens and a variety of chopped, diced, or shredded vegetables. Those who regard salads as "rabbit food" don't realize how many enriching nutrients and valuable enzymes they are missing.

Some of you may not be aware of the many different grains available. You can enjoy a different grain every day of the week and still look forward to those yet untried. Following is a list of whole grains to incorporate into your new diet: **brown rice, wild rice, corn and corn meal** (make sure these are organic or you run the risk of ingesting GMOs), **whole wheat, cracked wheat, bulgur wheat, pearl barley, barley flakes, hulled barley, whole rye berries, rye flakes, oatmeal, millet, quinoa, spelt, triticale, amaranth, teff, and kamut.**

Legumes consist of all varieties of beans and include lentils and green and yellow split peas. Each variety of beans sparks the taste buds with a very different flavor and texture. Since the digestive system may require a little time to adjust to the added fiber contained in legumes, begin with small amounts and increase slowly. Let your body be your guide to how much and how quickly to increase quantities.

If you are one who always thought of nuts as simply a snack, and one to be avoided because "they are too high in fat," reconsider them as an excellent source of protein. A handful or two a day are a good protein replacement. Though nuts are high in fats, they offer essential fatty acids so necessary to the body's many processes. Nuts are also delicious and add a delightful crunch to a dish.

Each kind of nut possesses different nutrients. You may have learned that one Brazil nut a day contains your daily requirement of selenium. Include seeds as well for their taste and health benefits. Following is a list of nut and seed varieties: **walnuts, *almonds, pecans, pistachios, hazelnuts, Brazil nuts, chestnuts, pine nuts, sunflower seeds, pumpkin seeds, sesame seeds, and flax seeds.**

Tofu, tempeh, and seitan are excellent ways to dress up a meal. Vegetarian cookbooks are a good source of information on how to prepare these foods and offer a myriad of creative soy food recipes. Tofu and tempeh are made from soybeans. Seitan, which may be less familiar to you, is made from wheat gluten.

There is no need to be concerned about getting enough protein on a vegetarian diet. High-protein foods such as tofu, tempeh, seitan, legumes, grains, and nuts and seeds are all easily obtainable and offer enough diversity to make vegetarian cooking fun and adventurous. Though they provide much smaller quantities, fruits and vegetables also contain protein.

Begin by serving one plant-based meal a week. Plant-based foods exclude animal products entirely. If this feels too drastic, begin by eliminating meat, chicken, and fish at that meal, but include dairy products. Refer to the list of **Comfort Foods** later in this chapter for ways to incorporate vegetarian foods without feeling that you are depriving yourself of the foods you enjoy. Serve your vegetarian meal with one or more steamed or cooked vegetables. Include a salad with a variety of fresh vegetables every day.

Then you progress to one full day of eating vegetarian. Begin your day with a whole-grain cereal, either cooked or dry. When shopping for your cereal, read the ingredient labels carefully and faithfully. Know what you're buying. Look for cereals that list "whole wheat flour," "whole rye flour," "whole barley flour, etc., rather than "wheat flour," "rye flour," etc.. Refined cereals are lacking vitamins and minerals that whole grains contain naturally. Look at the nutritional label. A true healthy cereal should have at least 5 g of fiber per serving. Include several pieces of fresh fruit throughout the day, every day.

It is very important to drink plenty of water. If possible, do your best to stay away from fluoridated water. Eliminate non-nutritional beverages, such as carbonated beverages and heavily sweetened juice drinks, and replace them with water preferably purified or distilled.

When you've succeeded with the whole vegetarian day, see if you can eliminate the animal-based foods at one meal every day. As you gain more confidence in your food preparation, establish new shopping directions, and as you realize the physical and emotional benefits you are enjoying, you will be encouraged to continue your new path.

For a truly healthy focus, one that will boost your energy and improve your mental skills, include a wide variety of foods every day. A plant-based diet consists of whole foods - foods that have their vitamins, minerals, phytochemicals, and enzymes intact - rather than extracted, refined, and rolled off the food factory lines in the little packages that cheat you out of nutrition. If, unfortunately, you choose to include eggs and dairy products in your vegetarian diet, you can consider these your source for protein. If you follow a vegan plan, include some items from each of the following categories each day to be assured of complete nutrition: Fruits, vegetables, grains, legumes, nuts and seeds.

Fruits

Enjoy several pieces of fruit each day. In fact, if you eat a piece of fruit before each meal and you're not yet on the vegetarian or vegan diet, that piece of fruit will cause you to eat less of what you are about to eat. It's a beginning.

Include many different fruits rather than concentrating on only one favorite fruit. One kind of fruit may not contain all the vitamins, minerals, phytochemicals, and enzymes your body needs.

Think variety by including the fruits of all colors. Each color contains different carotenes and different nutrients.

By all means consider purchasing certified organic fruits, for the increased vitamins and minerals they contain. Many fruits have skins that are completely edible and highly nutritious. Do not miss out on the opportunity to eat all the nutritious portions of a whole food.

Vegetables

Eat your veggies with abandon. You simply cannot over-consume vegetables. In fact, most people don't get enough.

Visit farmers' markets to get the best and freshest of the local vegetables that are in season. Most farmers pick their vegetables the day before and bring them to market early the following morning.

Experiment with vegetables that are new to you. Include some raw veggies each day. These contain enzymes that help the body's digestion, absorption, and elimination processes.

Your plate should include a mosaic of vegetable colors. Each color contains different phytochemicals in varying quantities. Phytochemicals are plant-based nutrients that benefit the body by strengthening the immune system to ward off diseases such as cancer and heart disease. We all have favorite foods, but rather than just eating broccoli or asparagus, try expanding your variety little by little to include some red vegetables, such as beets and tomatoes.

Include yellow vegetables, such as sweet potatoes and winter or summer squashes, and yellow bell peppers.

White vegetables include onions, turnips, cauliflower, parsnips and potatoes. Orange vegetables include carrots and rutabagas.

Green veggies are the largest group and include string beans, Brussels sprouts, artichokes, broccoli, asparagus, avocados, Swiss chard, cabbage, lettuces, and green bell peppers.

Include a fresh salad every day made with dark green lettuces, Russian kale, and lots of crunchy veggies. If you're only used to iceberg lettuce, it's time to take a walk on the wild side and try romaine, red leaf, green leaf, and any other variety you can find. These are higher in fiber and contain many more times the beta-carotene as iceberg lettuce.

Add a dressing that departs from those containing cheeses that overwhelm the flavor of the vegetables. Allow your taste buds to really enjoy the flavors of fresh veggies with extra virgin olive oil and a little balsamic vinegar, or a little oil and lemon juice. Better still; try to use an oil-free dressing.

Add some cooked veggies to your everyday meals, and introduce yourself to those that may be unfamiliar. Cook them only briefly or steam them to preserve their vitamins and minerals. Most veggies can be steamed, stir fried, and even roasted. Don't drown them in seasonings that cover up their wonderful flavor. Enjoy them in their natural state or with just a touch of seasoning.

Grains

Introduce whole grains into your diet. They contain bran that offers fiber and B vitamins, germ that provides essential fatty acids and vitamin E, and the endosperm that contains considerable protein.

Make your breakfast with whole-grain cereals such as oatmeal, Cream of Rye, quinoa flakes, barley flakes, cornmeal (organic), or buckwheat.

Sprinkle your cereal with raisins, dates, currents, nuts, sunflower seeds, pumpkin seeds, sesame seeds, maple syrup, honey, or date sugar. Then try using some vanilla soy milk or vanilla rice dream to top off your "breakfast sundae". The variety is endless. Whole-grain dry cereals are in abundance. Your local supermarket has some of these, but a natural foods store has the widest variety.

Read the ingredient labels carefully so you can make informed decisions. Look for cereals that contain at least 3 g of fiber per serving, preferably higher. Many whole-wheat cereals contain 5 or 6 g of fiber per serving.

Buy whole-grain breads rather than refined white breads. The whole-grain breads are higher in fiber and contain most of the B vitamins that have been processed out of the breads made with white flour.

Cook brown rice rather than white rice. Yes, it takes a bit longer to cook, but your health is worth more than the extra 20 or 30 minutes it takes to cook whole grains. Why not feed it to yourself directly rather than indirectly through the body of a dead animal?

Wild rice has a wonderful flavor, great texture, and 3 g of fiber per serving compared to 1 g of fiber for white rice.

Enjoy some whole-grain pastas instead of the usual refined pastas made of durum wheat. Natural foods stores sell pastas made from quinoa, spelt, rice, barley, buckwheat, and whole-wheat. The textures will be noticeably different, but these offer higher fiber content than durum wheat pasta.

Soak organic grains overnight and start them sprouting the next day. They should be ready for you within a day or two and can be added to a salad or sprinkled over almost any of your favorite foods.

Legumes

This category consists of all varieties of beans, including lent
and yellow split peas. Each type of bean has its own unique
flavor to lend variety to the vegetarian/vegan diet.

Beans can be easily incorporated into soups and salads, but don't stop
there. Put cooked beans into the food processor with seasonings and make
a dip. Mash beans with your favorite spices and make a sandwich spread
or even a sandwich filling. Try some new recipes that use beans as the
centerpiece of your meal; a vegetarian chili is one example. Beans are very
high in protein as well as vitamins and calcium.

Beans can be soaked overnight and put into a sprouting jar or bag
the next day. Within a day or two they should be ready to enjoy. Sprinkle
them over a salad or add them to soups or casseroles. Sprouted beans vastly
increase their vitamin and mineral content during the sprouting process.

Tofu, made from soybeans, provides almost unlimited creativity to
the vegetarian/vegan diet. Tofu comes in water-packed cartons and can be
found in most supermarkets. But, for organic varieties, shop at a natural
foods store.

Tofu is available in a number of different consistencies, including
regular, which is quite soft, to firm and extra firm varieties. The regular
tofu makes excellent sauces when prepared in a blender or food processor
with seasonings and spices. Firm and extra firm tofu work well in salads,
stir fries, or marinated and baked in the oven.

Delicious spreads that take the place of dairy products can be made in
the food processor by combining firm or extra firm tofu with seasonings
and by processing them to a smooth consistency.

Silken tofu comes in soft, firm, or extra firm and makes an excellent
base for savory sauces, fruity parfaits, or fruit smoothies. Many vegetarian
cookbooks include recipes for using tofu, while other cookbooks are devoted
completely to soy products.

Soy products abound these days and can be found in the form of veggie
hot dogs, lunchmeats, burger patties, ground "meat" style, veggie ham,
veggie fish, and veggie chicken. Many supermarkets sell these items

in the deli section. Natural foods stores offer a wider variety than most supermarkets. Asian markets will have some of the veggie meats in their freezer section. Be sure to read labels for ingredients, as some of these products may have ingredients you do not want to include in your diet, like MSG and its euphemisms.

Tempeh is a soy product that developed in Indonesia. It is made by fermenting soybeans in flat cakes. These offer further variety in the bean category and can be marinated, chopped, shredded, stir-fried, baked, or barbecued. Tempeh, an excellent source of protein, is available in natural food stores in the deli section or in Asian markets in the frozen food case.

Nuts

Nuts are a wonderful source of protein as well as essential fatty acids, fiber, and minerals. Nuts provide us with omega-3 and Omega-6 essential fatty acids that are important in the functioning of all the body's processes. Keep a variety of nuts on hand and store them in the refrigerator to avoid rancidity. Include walnuts, pecans, almonds, cashews, pistachios, hazelnuts, and Brazil nuts. Eat them in their raw state rather than roasted. The roasted nuts are roasted in oil, adding extra fats, which you may consider undesirable. In their raw state, nuts contain valuable essential fatty acids, which are lost when roasted or heated. Nuts add wonderful texture to a salad and can turn a pasta sauce into a special treat when added at the end of cooking.

Nut butters from organic sources are a delightful spread on apples and pears and enjoyed as a snack.

Nuts can be ground into a powder in a small electric coffee grinder. Add ground nuts to a sauce or a soup that needs a little thickening and boost the nutrition as well.

*Bear in mind that all almonds from California are irradiated due to contamination from an upwind slaughterhouse. Rather than do anything about the slaughterhouse, the California government irradiated the almonds.

Seeds

Seeds are a storehouse of protein, calcium, fiber, and essential fatty acids. Include pumpkin seeds, sunflower seeds, sesame seeds, and flax seeds. Since the seeds are very subject to rancidity, purchase them from a store that sells them in large quantities and turns them over quickly. Store seeds in the refrigerator to avoid rancidity. It is easy to incorporate seeds of all varieties into the diet.

Sesame seeds are delicious sprinkled on salads and over cereals. Sesame seed paste, also called tahini, makes a delicious sauce when mixed with lemon juice, garlic, water, salt, and a dash of cumin. This sauce enhances grain dishes, bean dishes, baked potatoes, and even pita sandwiches. Tahini can be also made into a salad dressing.

Sunflower seeds and pumpkin seeds add crunch to salads, cereals, and cooked grain dishes.

Flaxseeds can be ground in a small electric coffee grinder and sprinkled over cereals and salads for added fiber.

For sprouting, purchase organic seeds that are especially for sprouting use. They have not been sterilized and still contain the living germ. Try making your own alfalfa, red clover, radish, and onion seed sprouts. In their whole organic form, sunflower seeds are fun to sprout. It is a delight to see tiny sprouts emerging from their dark, tough, outer hulls.

Vitamin and Mineral Concerns

The term "vegan diet" may sound like a food regimen one might try temporarily as a weight loss plan or a regimen to regain one's health after an illness or trauma. While it brings success when applied for these purposes, a vegan diet is a lifestyle diet that, along with regular exercise, keeps one healthy and fit almost effortlessly.

To benefit fully from a vegan diet of plant-based foods, I suggest you familiarize yourself with a few concerns expressed by those unfamiliar with a well-planned program. I cannot emphasize enough the importance of including a wide variety of foods and consuming, on a daily basis, foods from each of the following groups: legumes, whole grains, fruits, vegetables, nuts and seeds.

Vitamin B12

The U.S. RDA (Recommended Daily Allowance) is 6 mcg. Since vitamin B12 is a cyanocobalamin, it is not readily available in a plant-based diet. It is important that you take a supplement to fulfill the body's needs. Actually, the best source of vitamin B12 is through **organic sulfur crystals** (see Chapter 19). Though the requirement seems small, this vitamin is essential to maintaining a healthy nervous system, important in preventing pernicious anemia, helpful in cell and blood formation, beneficial to proper digestion, fertility, growth, and necessary in the synthesis of DNA.

This vitamin is also an aid to people with menstrual difficulties, nervousness, insomnia, memory loss, depression, fatigue, skin problems, asthma, schizophrenia, and heart palpitations. If the label on the supplement says that it contains vitamin B12, make sure it includes the word cyanocobalamin or cobalamin. In this form the vitamin will be more readily absorbed.

Many foods are now fortified with vitamin B12. Look for it on soymilk labels, cereal packages, and meat and chicken substitutes made from soy protein.

The Red Star Company makes nutritional yeast in two varieties. Their Vegetarian Support Formula contains vitamin B12 as cyanocobalamin. Look for it in the natural food stores. Two heaping tablespoons a day will supply the needed RDA. Many new mothers find that it increases their milk production during lactation.

Calcium

The U.S. RDA is 1,000 mg. Calcium is an important mineral for maintaining firm bone structure and strong healthy teeth. This mineral helps us in other ways as well. It is essential for blood clotting, needed for muscle relaxation, permits regulation of cell metabolism, and helps nerve cell message transmission.

Maintaining healthy levels of calcium is rarely a problem on a well-planned vegan diet. You can find calcium in a multitude of plant foods. Vegetables that contain the highest calcium content include collards, kale, mustard greens, watercress, broccoli, okra, and dandelion greens. Sea vegetables such as wakame, arame, and dulse are also excellent sources of calcium. Many other foods in the plant kingdom contain rich stores of this vital mineral.

Impressive calcium content can be found in all legumes. Enjoy them daily for their exceptional calcium benefits. Within the bean family, soybeans rank highest in calcium, with navy beans and black beans following closely. Foods made from soybeans, such as soymilk, tofu processed with calcium, tempeh, and meat and chicken substitutes made from soy protein will provide plenty of calcium.

Nuts and seeds are good sources of this mineral, with almonds, hazelnuts and sesame seeds rating highest. Sesame tahini, added to salad dressings and sauces, is a good way to bring calcium into the diet.

Among the fruits, figs are tops for their calcium content. Oranges and fortified orange juice will deliver this mineral in ample quantities as well.

Vitamin D

The U.S. RDA is 400 IU. Vitamin D is technically a hormone that is manufactured in the skin when the skin is exposed to natural sunlight. Essential to our health, vitamin D helps the body to absorb calcium in order to maintain strong bones and teeth. Just 10 or 15 minutes a day of natural sun exposure will provide the body with enough vitamin D to function optimally. If you are unable to get direct sun exposure, look for foods fortified with this vitamin or take a supplement. Vitamin D can be absorbed through the eyes: from the eyes, to the retina, to the pituitary gland, and ultimately to strengthening the immune system.

When reading labels on fortified foods or supplements, vegans will want to choose those items labeled Vitamin D2 rather than Vitamin D3. Vitamin D2, or ergocalciferol, is synthesized from plant sources, mostly from yeasts through the process of irradiation. Animal sources, such as fish, sheep wool, hides, or cattle brains, provide the base for the manufacture of Vitamin D3.

Omega-3 fatty acids

Called essential fatty acids, these important fats perform many functions including enhancing the immune system, lowering cholesterol and triglycerides, preventing heart attacks, and reducing blood viscosity.

The Omega 3's are available from animal sources such as fatty fish and fish oil capsules; vegans can find sufficient quantities for many plant sources. Following are foods that contain ample quantities of Omega 3's: dark green leafy vegetables like kale and collards, broccoli, flax seed meal, flax seed oil, hemp seeds, hemp seed oil, soy beans, soy bean oil, firm tofu, walnuts, and walnut oil. Recommended daily servings of some items are as follows:

Flaxseed oil	1 teaspoon
Flaxseed meal	1 tablespoon
Walnuts	1/4 cup
Hemp seed oil	1 tablespoon
Soybeans	1 cup
Firm tofu	12 ounces

Iron

The U.S. RDA is 18 mg. An important mineral, Iron supplies oxygen to the cells throughout the body and carries away carbon dioxide as waste. It also helps immune system function and assists our mental processing.

Good sources of iron are found in all types of legumes and are especially high in soybeans and products made of soybeans, such as firm tofu. Grains are higher in iron, with quinoa ranking highest. Raw kale, raw spinach, mushrooms, and baked potatoes are also healthy sources.

Nuts and seeds are excellent sources of iron with pumpkin seeds, pine nuts, sesame seeds, and pistachios leading in quantities. Meat substitutes made from soy are outstanding sources for iron.

The iron content of blackstrap molasses is exceptionally high, making it an important source for this mineral.

Iron is best absorbed when eaten along with foods containing Vitamin C. Most vegetables qualify, as do citrus fruits. A little squeeze of lemon juice will easily enhance iron absorption.

Zinc

The U.S. RDA is 15 mg. A facilitator to many functions in the body, zinc wears many hats. A few of its many tasks include eliminating carbon dioxide, assisting wound healing, and helping the immune system.

Legumes are a good source of zinc, especially garbanzo beans and lentils. Products made from soy protein, such as the meat and chicken substitutes provide plenty of zinc. Wheat germ, millet, and quinoa being the highest among the grains, with all grains supplying healthy quantities.

Nuts and seeds offer ample zinc stores, with sesame tahini at the top of the list, followed by pumpkin seeds, cashews, and almonds.

Benefits of a Vegan Diet

If you were to prepare a health-oriented shopping list with specific goals you could aim for, your list might possibly look like this:

Normal blood pressure
Normal cholesterol
Clear, unclogged arteries
A trim figure
Plenty of energy
Sexual vitality
Pain-free days and nights
A good night's sleep
Good digestion
A sharp memory
Good concentration
A happy outlook

Do these goals seem like a fantasy or just plain wishful thinking? Actually, many nutrition-oriented doctors have learned through studies that lifestyle changes such as eating a plant-based diet, exercising and eliminating smoking, can help you attain these goals over time.

Because whole grains, legumes, fruits and vegetables are so high in complex carbohydrates, the body is supplied with plenty of energizing fuel. You won't have to drag yourself out for a walk - you will be bursting out the door willingly. Exercise tones the muscles, helps to maintain bone mass, and increases your levels of endorphins and hormones that heighten your sense of pleasure.

Whole grains contain many of the B vitamins that directly serve the nervous system. You may find yourself thinking more clearly, concentrating with more ease, maintaining a sharper memory, managing stress better, sleeping more soundly, and enjoying an overall feeling of well-being.

Certain foods have been beneficial in their ability to lower blood pressure. Some grains, such as oats and barley, and many varieties of beans, are noted for their soluble fiber that has helped to bring high blood pressure down to normal levels. The allium family, which includes onions and garlic, is also said to lower blood pressure.

All plant foods contain valuable phytochemicals that are known to protect the body from free radical damage. Free radicals are unstable oxygen molecules that damage our cells and are linked to a number of debilitating diseases, such as cancer, coronary artery disease, cataracts, and even aging.

Dr. Dean Ornish, and Dr. John McDougall, have seen evidence in their medical practices that a strict vegan diet reverses heart disease, lowers blood pressure, lowers cholesterol, and brings weight down naturally. The overall benefits you will derive from a vegan diet come from the increased intake of vitamins and minerals that help to strengthen the immune system, keep the bones strong, aid digestion, and bring excess weight down to normal.

The bonus benefit of a vegan diet is the ease of kitchen clean-up after preparing a hearty meal. Unless you are using an excess of cooking oils, plant-based foods are not naturally greasy. The pots and pans will not be greasy and the kitchen sink will not be greasy.

Are these attainable goals? Absolutely, but don't take my word for it. Try it and see for yourself. You have all to gain and nothing to lose.

COMFORT FOODS

Hamburgers

If you enjoy eating hamburgers, you can still enjoy burgers, but with a little tweaking of the ingredients. Use a whole-grain bun rather than one made of refined white flour. It is much more nutritious and it offers more fiber as well as richer flavor.

Fill your whole-grain bun with one of a variety of meatless burgers that are now available in many nationwide supermarkets in the frozen food case. Boca Burger makes a few different ones including one that is vegan. Gardenburgers come in different flavors including the vegan type. Morningstar Farms produces Hard Rock Cafe All Natural Veggie Burgers that are vegan patties. Worthington makes a fat-free vegan burger. My favorites are Amy's Sonoma or California burger as they are all organic and low fat. Add some fresh tomatoes, onions, lettuce and cucumber to your burger, and seek out a veggie mayonnaise such as Vegenaise, Nayonaise or Nasoya for the finishing touch on an incredible burger that won't clog up the arteries.

Check the frozen food case of your local supermarket as well as a natural food store for new products that appear with regularity. Recently some of the major food companies such as General Mills, Kellogg's, and Kraft have purchased companies that manufacture healthier foods. Vegetarian and vegan foods are easier to find than ever.

Pot Pies, Burritos, and Enchiladas

The brand called Amy's can be found in many supermarkets as well as Costco in the frozen food case. If the supermarket in your area does not carry this brand, check with your local natural foods store. Try requesting your local supermarket manager to order some vegetarian items. The markets want your business and will often honor requests.

Lunchmeats, Canadian bacon, Pepperoni

Yves Veggie Cuisine makes all of these and more. Veggie lunchmeats by Yves are made from soy products and wheat gluten and make for tasty sandwich fillings as well as great flavor additions to pasta sauces and casseroles. Find them in your natural foods store and some supermarkets. Request these products if your supermarket does not yet carry them.

Hot Dogs, Italian Links, Sausages

Yves, and Lightlife make their products from soy and wheat gluten with flavors that are difficult to distinguish from the real thing. These products are cooked and ready to heat and eat. Lightlife makes Gimmie Lean sausage, hot dogs, fake bacon, and more. Morningstar makes Veggie Dogs as well as Burgers.

With all these substitutes for anything that had a face and a mother, bear in mind that many of their spices are MSG euphemisms. So be very, very careful.

Chili

Fantastic Foods makes instant meals in a cup and is famous for their Cha-Cha Chili. They also make Chili Ole.

Bon appetite!

This article was reprinted with permission from Zel and Ruben Allen and can be found on their website - www.vegparadise.com - under the title *Vegetarian Basics 101*

Chapter 19

The Missing Essential Nutrient: Organic Sulfur Crystals

B ack in November of 2008, after I finished doing a radio show, I got in my car and was heading home. I turned on the radio to listen to the show that was on right after mine. It got my attention. They had a guest on the show who was talking about how his son, at the age of 16, was sent home to die with testicular cancer. The man then said that his son was then 27 years old and still alive. As I listened to the show and learned a little bit more about the substance that was used to cure his cancer, I figured that the stuff had to do with a lot more than just curing cancer. I was intrigued and I wanted to have this man as a guest on my show, but wasn't sure how to go about it. When I got home and went on my computer, there was an email from one of my listeners, Diane, who told me I should have the man as a guest on my radio show and supplied me with his telephone number. Fate works in strange ways!

The following Saturday, Patrick was a guest on my radio show. When the show was finished I could not believe that this stuff did everything he said it could. My history has always been that when a "magic bullet" comes along, I want to subject myself to it so I can tell my listeners that it's all a bunch of crap. So I ordered the product. In a mere 10 days, my energy level increased, and the asthma that I had since I was vaccinated as a child disappeared. Needless to say, it blew my mind. It's been over four years now that I've been taking this stuff and my asthma has not come back. Before I get into the benefits, let me give you a bit of back-story.

The product is known in the industry as methylsulfonymethane. It is sold and marketed very lucratively as MSM. The problem is, popular forms of MSM do not work because the original, natural product is bastardized. The process starts with crystals. The crystals are then turned into powder, which causes it to lose about 80% of its effectiveness. Then, anti-caking agents are added to it so it can be turned into pills. At this point, it is worthless! To derive the maximum benefits from MSM, it must be in its original crystal form, organic, and lignin or wood-based. The product I use and sell is harvested from the pine trees in Louisiana.

Organic sulfur is found in all living organisms. It is also contained in raw plant and animal foods. Organic sulfur is not found in any foods, which have been either destroyed during shipping, refrigeration, or cooking. Organic sulfur bonds with moisture and is therefore carried away when dehydration occurs - this is why stored, refrigerated, or cooked foods no longer contain organic sulfur.

With the introduction of the petro-chemical fertilizers in the 1930's, the benefits of sulfur were severely diminished and this is why you must stay hydrated and drink lots of water daily. Also, with the introduction of the petro-chemical fertilizers, which were created to replace manure as fertilizer and to create a cash crop for the petro-chemical industry, the oil-based fertilizers virtually destroyed all the sulfur in the soil. Add to this the obscene over-processing of our food supply (which served only to increase shelf life and profits and which made our food supply completely devoid of sulfur), it's no wonder that we are a nation of overweight, undernourished, disease-ridden 'sickos' hooked on pharmaceutical drugs.

In 1985, Finland became alarmed over the increasing and obscene disease rate of its population and abandoned all use of chemical fertilizers, fearing the levels of cadmium, yet totally unaware of the sulfur connection. Since doing so, they have become the leading supplier of organically grown foods in Europe. They have also seen their disease rates drop to 10% of their 1985 levels.

Interestingly enough, in 1985, the U.S. was at the same disease level as Finland. So, why did we not follow suit and ban the chemical fertilizers and put a lid on the highly processed foods? Well, as the theme song to Donald Trump's TV show begins: Money! Money! Money!

Do you really think that we could cease our use of profitable chemicals for our soil and our food, which involves commercial agribusiness, medicine, insurance, and genetic and designer foods? Maybe. But we could regenerate our own internal sulfur cycle with Organic Sulfur Crystals - provided that this product has not suffered the same indignities as our food supply.

In the body, Organic Sulfur (OS) is used to repair cells, which have been damaged, as well as to promote the growth of healthy new cells by allowing the cells to transport oxygen more efficiently. Organic Sulfur also makes cell walls more permeable, thus able to allow more nutrients in and to allow waste materials to pass out of the cells.

Studies have shown that fluorine is detrimental to such oxygen transport, yet this element has been added to our water supply to supposedly make our teeth healthier. Chlorine is also a detriment to the oxygen transport, but the amount in the water supply is inconsequential. These elements, however, are poisonous at higher concentrations and block the uptake of both oxygen and sulfur. To be safe, hook up a charcoal filter to your faucet and it removes the chlorine before you drink it. But like I said, a small amount of chlorine in the water has not been found to adversely affect the benefits of sulfur. If your water supply is fluoridated, try to get the best water filter money can buy to not have it in your system.

Every day the body uses up 750 mg of OS naturally. OS is natural and is actually found in the water we drink, as well as fresh, unrestored, and uncooked foods. It is found in fruits, vegetables, meat and dairy products. Unless you mostly consume organic raw foods, you are likely not receiving enough OS to realize its tremendous health benefits.

The benefits of OS are not only incredible, but are mind blowing as well.

OS has a cleansing or detoxifying effect on the cells within the body. It allows the body to remove toxins that have accumulated in all types of cells, including fat cells. When you begin this regimen, should you feel like you're getting the flu or other symptoms, understand that you are not getting sick. It is the detoxifying process and it will pass. While this is happening, DO NOT STOP TAKING THE CRYSTALS. The suggested usage is one teaspoonful twice a day - one in the morning and one in the evening. This can be done in several ways: dissolved in hot water, putting the crystals in your mouth and chewing them, dissolving them in hot water with a dash of lime, putting a tablespoon in a liter or a quart bottle, filling it with water and drinking it all day, or adding it to orange juice. Personally, I opt for the chewing method and then drink fresh orange juice. I've never tasted orange juice so sweet. One more thing - you can never take too much of the OS Crystals.

OS is not a drug or prescription medicine. It is actually a nutrient, or a food that the body can consume.

OS increases enzyme production within the glands of the body, substantially increasing the overall resistance to illness.

OS increases flexibility in the tissues within the body and increases blood circulation.

OS reduces muscle inflammation, promotes healing in the muscles, and prevents them from becoming sore. To the degree there is soreness, recovery and return to normality is quickened. Athletes, in particular, benefit from this as the intake of additional OS dramatically increases their recovery time.

OS eliminates so-called free radicals in the body. Allergies to pollens and certain foods can be reduced or eliminated by its use.

OS promotes healthy, increased growth of hair and fingernails.

OS has been studied for its anticancer effects. Because of the oxygenation of the cells and tissues, which creates an aerobic environment, cancer cells cannot exist.

OS studies have shown the reversal of osteoporosis, Alzheimer's disease, Parkinson's disease, and so far, 18 documented reversals of autism.

OS aids in healthy skin production and the reduction of wrinkles. It is one of the main ingredients in moisturizing cream.

OS helps the body properly regulate insulin production. Adequate OS in the diet can reduce the need for insulin injections.

OS helps in reducing and often eliminating diverticulitis. Parasites living in the colon are unable to remain attached to the colon walls on which OS forms a smooth, resistant coating. Hatching worms, have nothing to grab onto, and are flushed out.

OS helps to alleviate emphysema. It provides the body with material to manufacture new, healthy cells on lung walls.

OS, because of its ability to make cell walls more permeable, causes the body to rapidly release alcohol hangover toxins, removing them as waste from the body. The process happens far more rapidly than it normally takes to recover from a hangover, often as quickly as 20 minutes.

OS helps to alleviate chronic headaches. Increased circulation in the brain cells promotes proper blood circulation within the brain. Less pressure and pain result, reducing tendencies for headaches.

OS reduces hypoglycemia in the body because it has made it easier for the body to introduce blood sugar through more permeable cell walls. Less insulin is demanded for the process, resulting in less overuse of the pancreas. Several months of consistent OS usage can reduce or eliminate hypoglycemia entirely.

OS helps to alleviate PMS. To have more normal levels of production, OS enhances glandular production. Acid levels, enzyme levels, and hormonal levels are more evenly balanced with OS. Cramps, headaches, and nausea from the monthly cycle can be reduced or eliminated through OS usage.

OS helps to promote better kidney function more efficiently. Water retention problems due to bad kidney function can be alleviated.

OS can help alleviate eye problems. Dissolve 1 teaspoon of sulfur crystals in four ounces of water and use as eye drops as frequently as you like. We also have reports of astigmatism reversals within 3 years of taking the crystals.

OS will deliver essential omega-3 fatty acids throughout the body and will also allow the body to produce vitamin B12.

IMPORTANT: if you take any medication or supplements, there must be a 30 minute gap between the taking of the crystals and the taking of the meds and/or supplements. The synthetic chemicals and the anti-caking agents will nullify the benefits of the sulfur crystals.

There are many other benefits that the OS crystals provide. When I started taking the crystals in November of 2008, one of the listeners on my show was a candidate for heart bypass surgery. He was scared shitless and didn't want to go through that procedure so he ordered the crystals. One year later, he had no signs of needing bypass surgery. People on thyroid medication have eliminated or decreased their dosage. People with joint pain who had been taking MSM for years with no success reported the absence of pain within a week.

When things change, there is always a reaction or cause. From the petro-chemical fertilizers, which have made our soil incomplete for our sustainability, we have all gotten modern diseases. Do those who are lost in their minds, due to autism or Alzheimer's, come back when sugar is eliminated from their diets? No! But when sulfur is added to their diets, those that are lost, be they young or old, come back and remember who they are. Autism and Alzheimer's are both caused by vaccine delivered heavy metals, causing neurological disconnects. The sulfur, through its oxygen releasing abilities, enables the reconnects by sulfating the mercury, lead, aluminum and other adjuvants out of the blood brain barrier. And as Fukushima poses an imminent fall-out danger, sulfur can be used to protect and repair the damage of radiation exposure.

If you are interested in trying Organic Sulfur Crystals for yourself, please go to my website - www.healthtalkhawaii.com - and click on "Products and Services". As you scroll down a bit there is a little white box that has pricing information. Click on that white box and you will find prices, including postage for various parts of the world, for increments of two, four, and six containers. The crystals are sold in two 1-pound containers and last three months.

Chapter 20

Through the "Looking Glass

R ight now, despite all of our technological and scientific advances the world is inundated with violence. War, murder, theft, terrorism, abortion, child and spousal abuse are rampant. Since 1945, more than 140 wars have been fought and, in this country alone, an average of 16,000 people are murdered every year. Despite what we try to do to curb this, our solutions fail. Perhaps we should address the problem according to the law of karma and view the problem in accordance with the way we callously and brutally slaughter innocent and defenseless animals.

We live in an age that is virtually devoid of compassion. And, as inherent in the law of karma, every action has a reaction. If you kill or partake in killing, you will likewise be killed. So, how does the immense, unrestricted killing of animals come back to us? What about war? In this country, slaughterhouses and flesh centered restaurants are prolific. Additionally, every five or ten years there is a big war where multitudes are slaughtered even more cruelly than animals.

Spiritually, there is a difference between the body and the inhabitant of the body -- the soul. One is material, one is not. And, during the course of one's life, the living entity is encased within a particular type of body before evolving to another. Before that can happen they must finish the time they were allotted to remain in that body.

So, killing an animal or another living being that is not an aggressor, places an impediment in the completion of that cycle. If one kills simply to engage his senses in some sort of bizarre pleasure like feasting on flesh and blood, one incurs a reaction that must be paid for.

Basically, an animal, or fish, or bird, or whatever, must leave his body naturally. If not, the person (soul) in that body must come back in the same type of body and try again. This is the karmic restriction that is imposed upon him.

All these lower forms are evolving toward the human form. It is the human form that is the springboard to the spiritual world, to God's world. The laws of nature govern the lower forms. They do what they do instinctively and suffer no karmic reaction. The human form has a choice and, as previously mentioned, every action has a reaction.

If one lives like an animal, simply eating, sleeping, having sex and defending his turf, he does not differ from an animal. As such he takes birth in a lower form next time around and has to go through the evolving process to attain the human form again and again and again. The reaction to violence results in not only a waste of one's time in the material world, but also in the degradation of society as a whole. As if that weren't bad enough, everyone involved in the slaughter of those innocent animals, be it the one that owns the slaughterhouse, his workers, the waiter in the restaurant that serves the flesh and blood, the person that eats it, the housewife that prepares dinner, everyone and anyone has to take birth in that lower form for every hair that is on the creature's body. It will be a long time before they see the human form again.

The question always arises: aren't vegetables killed as well? To a degree, yes. Though the pulling of a mango off a tree is far less painful than slitting an animal's throat, there are two spiritual truths to consider. One, in Genesis the Lord says: "Behold, I have given you every seed-yielding plant that is on the surface of all the earth, and every tree which has fruit-yielding seed; it shall be food for you." And two, science has never been able to create a seed, which bears food. Only God has. As such, we offer our thanks to Him by offering plant foods to Him before we eat. He then takes that karmic reaction away from us, which in turn makes us more compassionate, caring, and aware. As corroboration of this, in the ancient eastern scripture, _Bhagavad-Gita As It Is_, the Lord says: "If one offers Me with love and devotion, a leaf, a flower, fruit or water, I will accept it." Nowhere does He suggest that we offer anything that had a face or a mother.

For those of you who do not believe in the transmigration of the soul or reincarnation, I refer you to Matthew in the New Testament where Jesus tells his disciples that John the Baptist appeared earlier and was known as

Elijah. He, Jesus, being the Son of God and fully enlightened, knew this. His disciples, still learning, did not.

Reference: Manusamhita, 5:51-52; Bhagavad-Gita As It Is, 9:26

Chapter 21

Recipes

Recipes contained herein are extremely simple and very easy to follow in making the transition from a flesh-based diet to a plant-based diet. Before the recipes though, I need to preface them with a piece of information.

I understand that for the most part the people I may be reaching are in a dietary transition phase of their lives. As such, I cannot be too hardcore in the recipes that I offer. Despite many recipes calling for olive oil, it is best to not use any added oils whatsoever to optimize a healthy quality of life.

For those of you trying to switch to a healthy diet for the first time, the elimination of added oils from your diet can come down the road after you have successfully abstained from eating anything that had a face or a mother, eggs and dairy products, for a comfortable period of time.

That being said: here goes!

BAKED "FRENCH FRIES"

Ingredients:

2 large potatoes

Extra light olive oil

Garlic powder

Turmeric powder

Onion Powder

Balsamic vinegar

Nutritional yeast

The How To:

Cut the potatoes into French-fry cut pieces.

Get a long Pyrex dish and pour a little extra virgin olive oil into the Pyrex dish. Next pour some of the oil into your hands.

Rub the oil all over the potato slices as you place them in the Pyrex dish always adding more olive oil to your hands as needed.

After all the potato slices are lined up in the Pyrex dish,

cover the potatoes with all the spices, adding the Balsamic vinegar at the end.

After this, cover all the potatoes with nutritional yeast, a huge source of B vitamins.

Bake for approximately 30 to 45 minutes making sure the potatoes are soft. For those of you who like French fries with mayonnaise, try Vegenaise instead. For those of you who are more traditional, ketchup works great.

To turn this dish into the "good ol' American meal", get a Sunshine South West, Barbeque or Breakfast burger, stick it in the toaster and put it on a burger bun with lettuce, tomato, cucumber, sprouts, ketchup and mustard and you will have one of the most filling and most satisfying meals ever.

YEAST TOAST

Ingredients:

2 slices of bread

Extra virgin olive oil

Nutritional yeast

Balsamic vinegar as an option

The How To:

Toast the bread

Cover with extra virgin olive oil and the Balsamic vinegar if you desire

Add the nutritional yeast.

It's that simple and it's loaded with B. vitamins.

GREEN SPLIT PEA SOUP

Ingredients:

2 cups green split peas

2 to 3 carrots

Onion

One package veggie, spicy Italian, sausage

Garlic powder

Curry powder

Cayenne or Sambal

Maple syrup

The How To:

It's best to soak the peas overnight. If you cannot, don't sweat it.

Put the split peas in a big pot and double or triple the amount of water.

Cut up the carrots and the onion, put them in the pot, add the spices and maple syrup to taste, and bring the water to a boil.

After the peas have gotten soft scoop them out and blend them. Put them back

in the pot, with the water, and cook for another half-hour.

Slice the veggie sausage and add to the soup.

Yummmy!

PASTA PRIMAVERA

Ingredients:

1 pound firm or extra firm tofu

Bragg's amino liquid

Extra light olive oil

White wine vinegar

1 cup fresh broccoli

1 or 2 cups asparagus spears

1 or 2 cups sweet peas

1 cup fresh mushrooms

1/2 cup chopped fresh parsley

1-1/2 tsp "Real Salt" (not the Morton's crap)

1/2 tsp garlic powder

1/4 tsp cayenne

sambal to taste

1 lb of angel hair pasta

The How To:

Cut the tofu into 2" X 1/2" X 1/8" pieces

Marinate the pieces for at least two hours in a mixture of 2 Tbsp Bragg's aminos,

1Tbsp extra light olive oil, and 2 Tbsp white wine vinegar.

After two hours brown the marinated tofu pieces lightly in 1 Tbsp extra light

olive oil and the leftover marinade, and set aside.

Boil until almost tender: 1 cup of fresh broccoli, the asparagus spears,

and the sweet peas. Drain and keep the liquid.

Sauté the mushrooms in 1Tbsp of extra light olive oil and set aside. Cook the pasta until tender and set aside.

But wait, there's more: the sauce.

Let bubble together gently over low heat for three minutes:

1/3 cup extra virgin olive oil and 1/3 cup unbleached white flour.

Whisk in, without making lumps, 3 cups of the set aside cooking water and the water

from the boiled veggies

Add the parsley, salt, garlic powder, cayenne, and Sambal.

Continue cooking over low heat until thickened and smooth. Then add the tofu, veggies and mushrooms to the sauce, and serve over the pasta.

"MEET" LOAF

Ingredients:

1 pound firm or extra firm tofu

1/2 cup wheat germ

1/3 cup parsley

1/4 cup onion, chopped, or 1 Tbsp onion powder

2 Tbsp Bragg's amino liquid

2 Tbsp nutritional yeast

1/2 Tbsp Dijon mustard

1/4 tsp garlic powder

1/4 tsp black pepper

1/4 cup tomato ketchup

The How To:

Mix everything together except the ketchup and parsley.

Oil a loaf pan or Pyrex dish with 2 Tbsp extra virgin oil.

Press the tofu mixture into the oil loaf pan and bake for about an hour.

Let cool about 10 minutes before removing from the pan.

Garnish with ketchup and parsley.

It's also good sliced and/or fried for sandwiches the next day.

TOFU FRIED RICE

Ingredients:

4 cups cooked brown, wild blend, or Basmati rice

1 Tbsp extra light olive oil

4 cloves of garlic, crushed

1 cup chopped green onions

1 lb tofu

Bragg's amino liquid

1-1/2 cups onion, diced

1 cup celery, diced

1-1/2 cups bean sprouts

1/2 bag of frozen veggies (carrots, peas, corn)

Sambal hot sauce

The How To:

Cook and have ready 4 cups of the cooked rice.

Heat in a heavy skillet or wok: 1 Tbsp olive oil and 2 cloves of crushed garlic.

Cook until garlic is light brown, then remove and discard the garlic.

Add and stir-fry the tofu, diced, for 1 minute.

Add and stir-in well the Bragg's.

Remove the tofu from the pan.

Add to the pan: diced onion and celery and stir-fry for 2 - 3 minutes.

Add the cooked rice and stir-fry until all mixed.

Add the fried tofu, bean sprouts and veggies.

Stir-fry 2 minutes, then add another Tbsp Bragg's and Sambal to taste.

Mix well and serve hot, topped with the green onions.

MOCK CHICKEN NUGGETS

After you have made this once you will get creative. It's great hot or served cold in a salad.

You can make it with BBQ sauce, teriyaki sauce, peanut sauce, or sweet & sour sauce.

Ingredients:

1 block firm tofu drained well.

3 Tbsp light olive oil

3 Tbsp Bragg's amino liquid

1/3 cup nutritional yeast

1/4 tsp black pepper

1 tsp garlic powder

The How To:

Drain the tofu well and cut into cubes.

Heat oil in a frying pan.

When hot, add the tofu and cook for about 5 minutes before turning. This allows the tofu to brown.

When evenly browned turn off the heat and add the remaining ingredients and stir until evenly coated.

Serve with brown rice and increase the protein content by 4 times.

BEANLESS, DAIRYLESS ENCHILADAS

Ingredients:

1 block firm tofu, drained well.

Pasta sauce.

Veggies like: carrot, onion, zucchini, red and green bell peppers

Spices like: oregano, garlic powder, basil, thyme, curry powder, etc.

Bragg's amino liquid

Light olive oil

Nutritional yeast

Organic corn tortillas

Honey

The How To:

Preheat the oven to 350 degrees.

Heat up the pasta sauce in whatever you heat up pasta sauce in. When hot, add a bit of honey to offset the acidity of the tomatoes.

Cut the veggies small, put in a separate pot, add some water and some spices and cook until soft.

Cut the tofu in small pieces and fry with some olive oil, Bragg's and the other spices until brown.

When the veggies and tofu are done, combine them.

Cover the bottom of a baking pan with some pasta sauce.

Fill a tortilla with the veggies and tofu and put it, fold down, in the baking dish.

Do this with all the tortillas. When they are lined up cover them with pasta sauce, but do not use all the sauce.

Combine the remaining pasta sauce, veggies and tofu and cover the tortillas with them.

Cover everything with nutritional yeast and bake until really soft. Maybe 15 - 20 minutes.

"Betcha can't eat one!"

PAELLA

Paella is the world's most famous rice dish from Spain. It is cooked in a typical stainless steel paella pan, and the rice used is the original Bomba rice. It is an ancient strain of rice grown in the area of Bomba, Spain. In this recipe you can substitute the Bomba rice with Arborio, Basmati, or brown rice, which are available at most natural food stores.

Ingredients:

1/3 cup light olive oil

1 small onion

2-3 garlic cloves, crushed

3-5 Tbsp minced fresh parsley

1 tsp saffron

1 cube GMO & MSG-free vegetable bouillon

1 pkg veggie meat nuggets

1 medium green bell pepper, sliced

1 medium red bell pepper, sliced

8 oz tomato sauce

4 cups pre-cooked rice

7 cups water

1/2 tsp sambal or hot sauce, to taste

The How To:

Sauté onion, parsley and garlic until the onion becomes transparent.

Add saffron, bouillon, veggie meat nuggets, and peppers until the nuggets are slightly browned.

Add the tomato sauce and stir (add a bit of honey to offset the acidity.)

Add rice and water and bring to a boil.

Transfer to a baking dish and bake at 325 degrees for 15-20 minutes.

CHINESE SWEET & SOUR BALLS

Ingredients:

First, pre-heat your oven to 350 degrees

1Tbsp peanut butter

1 Tbsp Bragg's aminos

1 block firm tofu

1/2 cup whole wheat flour

1/2 cup green bell peppers

1/4 cup sliced fresh mushrooms

1/4 cup sliced fresh celery

4 green onions, sliced thin

The How To:

Whip together the peanut butter and Bragg's.

Mash the tofu in a bowl.

Mix everything in with the tofu.

Form into 1-1/2 " balls, then arrange them in a Pyrex baking dish.

(It would be good to spread a bit of light olive oil on the bottom of the Pyrex dish so they don't stick.)

Bake for 20 minutes, then carefully turn each ball over and bake for another 20 minutes.

Serve on rice with sweet & sour sauce, which you can buy or make. See below.

Sweet & Sour Sauce

Combine in a saucepan over medium heat:

1 cup unsweetened pineapple juice

6 tbsp sweetener of your choice - maple syrup or honey

6 Tbsp Bragg's apple cider vinegar

2 Tbsp Bragg's aminos

1 1/2 Tbsp cornstarch

1/4 tsp garlic powder

Then whisk out all the lumps and heat and stir constantly until thickened.

SWEET & SOUR TOFU

Ingredients:

First, pre-heat your oven to 350 degrees

Light olive oil

1 lb firm tofu

1/2 cup cornstarch

1/4 cup (non GMO & MSG) vegetable bouillon broth

2 Tbsp Bragg's aminos

The How To:

Cut the tofu into cubes.

Deep-fry the tofu cubes in heated oil being sure the cubes stay separate in the oil;.

Remove when golden brown (about 3 - 5 minutes).

Drain and serve with sweet & sour sauce. (See above)

SPAGHETTI BALLS

First, pre-heat your oven to 350 degrees

Ingredients:

1 lb firm tofu mashed

1 Tbsp onion powder

1/2 cup wheat germ

1/4 cup chopped parsley

2 Tbsp Bragg's aminos

2 Tbsp nutritional yeast

1/2 tsp garlic powder

1/4 tsp black pepper

1/4 tsp oregano

a bit of light olive oil

The How To:

Spread a baking pan with some light olive oil.

Form the mixture into 1-1/2 " balls and arrange in the pan.

Bake about 30 minutes carefully turning the balls around every 10 minutes until browned.

(It's called "Spaghetti Balls" because we use Italian food spices).

INDONESIAN SATAY

Because you must marinate the tofu you'll need to start this about 2 hours or more before you plan to eat.

Ingredients:

2 cloves garlic

1" cube fresh ginger root peeled

1/4 cup boiling water

2 Tbsp Bragg's aminos

2 Tbsp peanut butter

2 tsp honey or maple syrup

1/2 tsp ground coriander

1/8 tsp cayenne

1/2 tsp Bragg's apple cider vinegar

1 lb firm tofu cut into 1/2" slices

The How To:

In Pyrex dish put a bit of olive oil on the surface.

Process all the ingredients, except the tofu, in a food processor, blender, etc. until smooth.

Put a thin layer of the blend into the Pyrex dish.

Arrange the tofu slices in a single layer.

Pour the rest of the mix over the tofu.

Marinate for an hour or two.

bake at 350 degrees for about 45 minutes.

Serve with rice and a salad.

INDONESIAN GADO GADO

Can be served warm or cold with rice or quinoa.

Ingredients:

9 oz Chinese bok choy

cut into small pieces

4-1/2 oz mung bean sprouts

4-5 small potatoes cooked

1 cup string beans, topped & tailed

1 lb firm tofu, cubed

3/4 cup raw peanuts

4 - 5 Brazil nuts

1tsp chili powder

1 cup cold water

1tsp Sambal

1/2 tsp onion powder

1/2 tsp garlic powder

1 tsp honey or maple syrup

1 Tbsp Bragg's aminos

1/2 cup coconut milk

1 medium cucumber, sliced

1small bunch watercress

1 Tbsp fresh lemon juice

The How To:

Blanch the bok choy leaves in boiling water for 1 minute and drain.

Blanch the bean sprouts in boiling water for 30 seconds and drain.

Cook the bite-sized potatoes in boiling water.

Deep-fry the tofu until slightly golden. Add the Bragg's.

Cook the string beans in boiling water for 5 minutes and drain.

Deep-fry the peanuts until golden and remove.

Deep-fry the Brazil nuts until golden and remove.

Blend until smooth the chili powder, onion and garlic powder, fried nuts and sweetener.

Add the 1 cup of cold water to the mix.

Transfer the contents to a large frying pan, bring to a boil and stir for 10 minutes.

Add the coconut milk and lemon juice and remove from the heat.

Pile the Chinese bok choy, bean sprouts, potatoes, beans, tofu, cucumber and watercress in individual piles on a large serving dish and immediately pour the dressing over the salad and serve.

The dressing may also be served separately.

KOREAN BBQ TOFU

Ingredients:

1-1/2 lbs firm tofu

1/2 cup Bragg's aminos

6 Tbsp sweetener (maple syrup, preferably)

1 tsp dry mustard

4 cloves garlic or 1/2 tsp garlic powder

2 tsp onion powder

1 to 2 Tbsp light olive oil

green onions

mushrooms

snow peas

rice

The How To:

Cut the tofu into 1/4" slices

Marinate for at least 2 hours (overnight is best) in a mixture of:

Bragg's, sweetener, mustard powder, garlic, onion powder

After marinating, brown on both sides and serve with a garnish of the chopped green onions, mushrooms, and snow peas.

Serve over rice.

FILET DE TOFU

Ingredients

2 lbs firm tofu

1 tsp paprika

2 Tbsp minced parsley

1 tsp chives, chopped fine

1 tsp real salt

1/2 tsp black pepper

1-1/2 cup vegetable bouillon

Nori or other seaweed

lemon

The How To:

Preheat your oven to 350 degrees

Boil the tofu slices in salted water for 20 minutes with the seaweed added

Drain and let cool

In a Pyrex baking dish or a baking pan

lay the slices close together and sprinkle with the paprika, parsley, chives, and black pepper

Carefully pour the bouillon - about 3/4 cup - in and around the tofu pieces without disturbing the herbs and spices

Bake for 20 minutes or until almost all the liquid is gone

Remove pan from oven and pour the rest of the liquid on in the same way as before.

Bake another 10 minutes until liquid is almost gone again.

Brush with extra virgin olive oil

Squeeze on fresh lemon to taste.

Then broil until lightly browned and serve with the parsley garnish

BETTER 'N SCRAMBLED EGGS

This recipe's heading speaks for itself. Instead of the high cholesterol omelet or scrambled eggs

simply replace the eggs with a block of tofu and some spices to get a better tasting substitute!

Ingredients:

1 block tofu

1 Tbsp light olive oil

1/4 tsp maple syrup

1 onion chopped

1 tsp turmeric

1 Tbsp Bragg's aminos

1 tsp garlic powder 1/2 tsp Cajun spice (if you can find it)

Vegetarian "sausage" or vegetarian "Canadian bacon"

The How To:

Fry the onion in the light olive oil until the onion turns transparent.

Crumble the tofu into the pan and add the spices.

Cook until done, stirring frequently.

Fry up the sausage or bacon and serve.

For a more "Spanish style" omelet, add tomato, red, green and yellow bell peppers and some cooked potatoes to the mix and then top with some salsa.

MOCK TURKEY PATTIES

Ingredients:

1 block firm tofu

1/2 cup Bragg's amino

1 tsp poultry seasoning

1/2 cup nutritional yeast

1/4 cup whole wheat flour

some black pepper

The How To:

Preheat the oven to 350 degrees

Cut the tofu into slices

Mix the nutritional yeast, poultry seasoning and whole-wheat flour together

Dip each slice of tofu in the Bragg's then into the breading mixture

Place on a lightly oiled baking sheet and bake for 15 minutes

Turn the tofu over and bake for another 15 minutes until a light golden brown

Serve the slices with holiday gravy

HOLIDAY GRAVY

Ingredients:

1/4 cup light olive oil

1 cup garbanzo flour (chickpea)

1 tsp basil\1/2 tsp thyme

1/2 tsp black pepper

3 cups water

1/4 cup Bragg's

2 tsp lemon juice

2-3 Tbsp nutritional yeast

The How To:

Combine first 5 ingredients, stirring constantly over medium-high flame until lightly toasted. You may have to mash it with the backside of the spoon. When toasted, gradually add water, stirring constantly to prevent lumping (whisking is ideal). When blended, add last ingredient and mix well. Makes about 1 quart.

SPICY PEANUT PASTA

Ingredients:

8 oz pasta shells

1 large carrot

2 cups broccoli florets

2 green onions, sliced

1 medium green bell pepper, sliced

1/2 cup creamy peanut sauce (below)

2 Tbsp chopped peanuts

The How To:

Cook the pasta.

Steam the carrots and broccoli for 3-5 minutes.

Mix green peppers, steamed veggies and creamy peanut sauce in a pan over low heat.

Drain pasta and add to vegetable mixture with green onions and mix thoroughly.

Garnish with chopped peanuts.

CREAMY PEANUT SAUCE

Ingredients:

1/4 cup peanut butter

1/4 cup plain non-fat yogurt or eggless mayonnaise

1 garlic clove, minced

1tsp sweetener

1 tsp Bragg's amino

1/4 tsp dark sesame oil

1/2 tsp ground ginger

1/4 tsp crushed red peppers

1 tsp hot water

The How To:

Combine all ingredients in a mixing bowl and mix with a whisk.

makes about 1/2 cup of peanut (satay) sauce

CHRISTMAS STUFFING

Ingredients:

2 cups whole grain bread crumbs

1/2 cup cooked lentils

1/2 cup chopped walnuts

2-3 Tbsp light olive oil

1/2 cup diced celery

1/2 cup diced onion

1/2 cup blended tomatoes

1 tsp ground sage

1/2 tsp thyme

1/2 tsp raisins

2 Tbsp arrowroot mixed in 1/4 cup water

olive oil for basting

The How To:

Preheat oven to 350 degrees and oil a loaf pan. Combine the first 3 ingredients and cook for about 5 minutes.

Add the next 3 ingredients and stir constantly until thickened. Pour into the mixture of dry ingredients. Place

in an oiled loaf pan and bake at 350 degrees for about an hour. Baste the top every 15 minutes with light olive oil.

TOFU CHICKEN HEKKA

Ingredients:

1 block tofu

2 oz long rice

3 Tbsp light olive oil

1 onion, cut in half-moon slices

1/2 cup julienne carrot

1 clove garlic, minced

1/2 cup julienne celery

1 Tbsp chopped ginger

1/2 cup sliced bamboo shoots

4 fresh shitake mushrooms, sliced

1/2 lb watercress cut into small pieces

4 green onions cut small

Sauce:

1/3 cup dry sweetener

1/2 cup Bragg's

1/2 cup mock chicken broth

2 Tbsp cooking wine

The How To:

Break the tofu into 1 inch squares, place on lightly oiled baking pan, sprinkle with Bragg's and bake until brown (3/4 hour at 350).

Combine ingredients for sauce. Soak long rice in warm water for 10 minutes, then drain and cut smaller. Heat remaining oil and cook onion until translucent. Add carrot and celery and stir-fry for 2 minutes. Add garlic and stir-fry 1 more minute. Add sauce, tofu, long rice,

bamboo shoots and shitake mushrooms to skillet and simmer for 5 minutes. Add green onions and heat through, about 5 minutes. Serve with steamed rice.

BREAKFAST BURRITOS

Ingredients:

1 tsp light olive oil

1 small onion

3 Tbsp roasted green chilies, diced

1/2 cup tomatoes, chopped

2 medium potatoes, cooked and chopped

1 lb soft tofu, mashed

1/2 tsp garlic powder

1/2 tsp oregano

1/2 tsp cumin powder

1/2 tsp turmeric

1 tsp real salt

4 large or 8 small whole-wheat tortillas 1/2 cup salsa

4 oz non-dairy cheese (optional)

The How To:

Heat oil in skillet and saute' onions until translucent. Add green chilies, tomatoes and potatoes, and saute' 5 minutes.

Stir in mashed tofu, garlic, oregano, cumin, turmeric and salt. Cook on low heat 5 minutes. Add grated cheese, if used, and set aside.

To warm tortillas, dry cook them in a skillet for a few minutes on each side.

Portion tofu-potato mixture according to number of tortillas and spoon portions into center of each tortilla. Spread 2 Tbsp salsa across filling.

Fold in the edges and roll up burrito-style. Serve with additional salsa on the side.

PAGHETTI, FAST & EASY

Ingredients:

Morningstar, Boca Burger or Yves Veggie "Ground Beef"

1/2 pkg. whole grain spaghetti or angel hair pasta

sliced mushrooms

1 chopped onion

1 chopped tomato

1 tsp cinnamon

1 tsp lemon juice

hot sauce

garlic powder

1-2 Tbsp Bragg's aminos

spaghetti sauce or salsa

light olive oil

The How To:

Cook the spaghetti or angel hair pasta about 5 minutes and let it sit in the water so it doesn't get hard and stick together.

In a skillet, fry the onion and mushrooms in a bit of the olive oil until the onions are glazed and the mushrooms done.

Then add the chopped tomato.

After a couple of minutes add the veggie "ground beef", cinnamon, lemon juice, hot sauce, garlic powder and the Bragg's.

Let this saute for a bit and before it gets dry add the pasta sauce or salsa.

Put this on top of the pasta and serve with a green salad and French bread.

EGGLESS EGG SALAD

Great taste without the high cholesterol and high fat. It's so easy to make and you can make a large batch and keep it in the fridge for sandwiches on pita bread, or whatever, and as a snack or a last minute meal.

Ingredients:

1/2 cup tofu, drained

1 tsp Bragg's

1 tsp Dijon mustard

2 tsp Vegenaise

1 tsp nutritional yeast

1 Tbsp green onions, finely diced

2 Tbsp grated carrots

1 Tbsp celery, finely diced

1 Tbsp fresh parsley, minced

1 tsp turmeric

1/2 tsp black pepper

1/2 tsp garlic powder

The How To:

Mash the tofu with a fork.

Stir in all the ingredients and mix well.

For a great sandwich, use pita bread and add some lettuce, tomato, onion, cucumber, and a touch of sweet chili sauce.

CURRY VEGGIES

Ingredients:

2 cups cubed potatoes

1 cup cubed carrots

1 can garbanzo beans

1 cup chopped onions

1 cup peas

1 cup broccoli heads

1 cup cauliflower heads

1 cup snow peas

1 cup mushrooms

1 cup water

3 tsp mild curry paste

1 can coconut milk

1/2 tsp real salt

1 tsp garlic powder

1 Tbsp Bragg's

1 Tbsp light olive oil

1 block cubed firm tofu

The How To:

Heat the oil in a large saucepan on medium high heat.

Add the onion and saute for a minute.

Add the potatoes, carrots, broccoli and cauliflower.

Add the water and boil until the potatoes start to get soft.

Add the coconut milk, real salt, curry paste, peas, garbanzo beans, mushrooms and snow peas.

Let simmer until the veggies are cooked.

Sprinkle with the garlic powder and Bragg's and fry until golden brown.

Add the cubed tofu at the end, cook for another minute or so stirring constantly and serve with sticky, Basmati, wild, or brown rice.

PIZZA, PIZZA

Ain't nothin' in the world like a "do-it-yourself" pizza. The hassle, though, has always been the crust. Enter the Alvarado, California-style pizza crust, which you can get from your local natural food store in the frozen section. They make a low-fat and an original. The difference is that the original contains dairy products, the low-fat is vegan, and both contain only all-natural ingredients.

My Favorite Ingredients:

Spicy salsa or tomato sauce

Garlic Powder

Curry powder

Turmeric

Hot sauce

Cut in small pieces:

Onions

Mushrooms

Broccoli

Red and green bell peppers

Optional:

Veggie pepperoni

Veggie ground beef

Veggie sausage

The How To:

Cover the crust with the salsa or tomato sauce.

Then add the spices and then the veggies and then the veggie "meats".

Preheat the oven to 350 degrees (remember, anything higher creates cancer-causing acrylimides).

Put the pizza on a baking tray and heat for about 25 minutes.

Yeah, yeah, you non-vegans can add cheese if need be.

MASHED POTATOES & SAUERKRAUT, GERMAN STYLE

Ingredients:

2 large potatoes

1 large sweet onion

1 package veggie sausage

1 jar sauerkraut

1/4 cup non-canola oil rice milk

1 tsp real salt

1 tsp extra light olive oil

potato masher

The How To:

Boil the potatoes until soft

Pour off the water

Add salt and rice milk

Mash until smooth

Mix in the sauerkraut

Lightly brown the onion and sausage

Add to the potatoes and mix well.

SIMPLE SPUDS

Ingredients:

Potatoes and/or sweet potatoes (quantity will vary in accordance with your appetite)

Vegenaise (Follow Your Heart - reduced fat)

Salsa

The How To:

Cut the potatoes into medium sized pieces and steam them

(This can be done by placing a steamer basket into a saucepan with water and heating over medium to high heat until the potatoes are soft)

Put potatoes into a bowl and add some Vegenaise and salsa to taste

It's that simple!

PORTABELLA PILAF

Ingredients:

Portobello mushrooms to meet the number of people to serve

1 cup quinoa

2 cups water

Light olive oil

Spicy barbeque sauce

Maple syrup

Nutritional yeast

Cayenne (to taste)

Garlic powder (to taste)

Cumin (to taste)

Turmeric (to taste)

1 small onion

1 sweet potato

1 small red and green bell pepper

1 zucchini

The How To:

Cut the veggies into small pieces

Start cooking the quinoa

Add the veggies and the spices to the cooking quinoa

When cooked, add nutritional yeast, stir well and let stand

Remove stems from the mushrooms

Place mushrooms on a lightly oiled baking pan

Brush barbeque sauce on the mushrooms

Scoop quinoa and veggies and place on the mushrooms

Drizzle maple syrup on the quinoa

Bake at 350 degrees for about 20-30 minutes

ENERGY SHAKE

Ingredients:

4-5 cups of water, to soak

1 cup raw, hulled sunflower seeds

1/3 cup raw almonds (not from California)

2/3 cup raisins

1/2 cup carob powder

1/4 cup honey

4 heaping Tbsp non-GMO lecithin granules

2 tsp grain coffee-substitute

The How To:

Soak the first 4 ingredients together for 24 hours

Pour the 4 ingredients into a blender and add the rest

Blend until smooth

Serve as is or with fresh fruit or whole grain toast or toasted bagel

BREAKFAST SHAKE

Ingredients:

2 cups carob Rice Dream (or more according to taste)

2 large frozen bananas

1/2 cup organic strawberries

1/2 cup organic blueberries

1 tsp maple syrup

1/2 cup ice cubes

Blend until smooth

Serve as is or with whole grain toast or toasted bagel

THE "BIG KAHUNA" ACAI BOWL

Ingredients:

Sambazon pure unsweetened Acai (sold as "smoothie packs") Select 'unsweetened' rather than the other options because the others contain enormous amounts of caffeine

Frozen bananas

Frozen organic strawberries

Frozen blueberries or the Costco organic berry mix, containing blueberries, blackberries and raspberries.

Fresh bananas

Fresh organic strawberries

Fresh organic blueberries

Fresh organic raspberries

(I emphasize organic because all berries are otherwise heavily pesticided)

Honey

Bee pollen

Your favorite granola (i.e.: hemp granola)

Vanilla Rice Milk or organic vanilla soymilk

The How To:

In a blender (preferably a Vita Mix), place the frozen ingredients plus the liquid to cover 3/4 of the frozen ingredients.

Blend until smooth.

Place some granola on the bottom of a bowl and add the blended mix with some honey on the top.

On top of that add more granola.

On top of that add banana slices and all the fresh berries.

Top off with bee pollen.

As they say in Hawaii, "Da bugga broke da mout!"

THE "BEATS ALL" BURGER

Before I get into talking about the burger, I need to preface it with this. We all know there's nothing that beats a dynamite burger. However, the problem we're faced with is FAT. But what if you could eat a burger that was low in fat, healthy and incredibly satisfies your pallet? Bear in mind that this is my choice. So, if need be, get creative. Here goes!

Ingredients:

Amy's Sonoma burger (all organic and made with quinoa)

French Meadow Bakery Certified Organic 100% Rye Bread with Sunflower seeds

Lettuce

Tomato

Sprouts

Onion

Cucumber

Avocado

Hummus

Ketchup

The How To:

Put the burger, which is pre-cooked in the toaster, at full heat.

Toast the rye bread until crunchy

Put avocado on one of the slices of bread

Put hummus on the other slice of bread (see hummus recipe below)

Start layering on one of the slices:

Tomato

Cucumber

Onion

Burger

Ketchup

Lettuce

Sprouts

Cover with the other slice

Remember that this is my personal preference. So, if you want to fry the onions or fry mushrooms or whatever, there are no hard and fast rules.

HUMMUS

For this to work you will need either a Vita Mix or a Blend Tech blender. Also, when you get the hang of it, there are no hard and fast rules. So, anything goes.

Ingredients:

A 25 oz can of garbanzo beans or

Two 15 oz cans of garbanzo beans or

Soak 25 – 30 ounces of garbanzo beans until they double in size

(probably a day or two)

Tomato

Onion

Garlic powder

Seseme Tahini

Lemon

Chipolte Spice

Maple Syrup

Bragg's Liquid Aminos

Water from the garbanzo beans

The How To:

First put in the lemon

Then the veggies,

Spices

Syrup

Beans

Then blend, stop and stir, and continue blending, repeating the process until you get the consistency you want.

After it's done, put it in a container and refrigerate. You can use the hummus as a salad dressing, on carrot or celery slices or whatever.

Chapter 22

At The Water Hole

You all know that old expression, "You can lead a horse to water but you can't make him drink." If you share my opinion, here you are!

From what you have read in this book, I hope you can see the sanity of a vegan diet centered on organic whole grains, organic fruits and vegetables, organic beans and legumes, organic nuts and seeds, fresh juices, and superfoods. You have read about the ills of artificial sweeteners, genetically modified foods, excess sugar, and pasteurized dairy products. You have learned that all sources of nutrition can come from plant foods and that flesh foods are not at all necessary. You have read that simply by changing your diet you can reverse so many degenerative diseases and eliminate the need for prescription medications.

Although conditioning has dictated to you a path that may be difficult to walk away from, a dietary change is something that you must do in order to prolong your life, to be healthy, alert, and free of pain and disease.

The insanity of this world can best be found in an article that was written by the "Health Ranger," Mike Adams, at his website, www.naturalnews. com. His satirical article of November 1, 2010, *'Diabetes rises 1% among U.S. children and teens following Halloween candy blitz'*, says:

"Diabetes rose 1% among United States children and teens yesterday as tens of millions of households handed out literally thousands of tons of candies made with refined white sugar and High Fructose Corn Syrup (HFCS). The event, of course, is called 'Halloween,' and each year it subjects tens of millions of children to artificial food coloring chemicals and refined sugars that promote diabetes and obesity - diseases that ultimately lead to death."

The "one percent" number is just an estimate, of course. But here is a statistical fact: **One-third of US adults will have diabetes by 2050** (unless something drastic changes). That's the conclusion of a recent CDC report that looked at the progression of the disease.

Given that America is headed towards a **diabetes pandemic,** is it really such a great idea to have a holiday each year that involves handing out diabetes promoting candies to children and teens? If the country were suffering from an out-of-control alcoholism pandemic, would it make sense for homes to hand out free booze?

What is Halloween really celebrating?

There are better ways to celebrate Halloween, it would seem, than distributing highly addictive sugars and food coloring chemicals, to children who are already overdosing on processed foods. But what is Halloween celebrating in the first place?

What kind of holiday sees families erecting what appears to be **dead bodies** in their front yards? What kind of holiday worships demons, zombies and ghouls? What kind of weird, warped message does it send to children when you entice them with bag loads of candy while surrounding them with images of witches, skeletons, blood and death?

It almost seems like some sort of sick psy-ops agenda. And yet parents just go right along with it, without even questioning (for the most part) what their children are eating.

Sure, it's great to see children being creative with fun costumes and social interaction with other kids. That's the good side of Halloween. But the ugly side, with all the toxic candy and graphic, bloody imagery is pretty darned ugly. It's not only bad for children's bodies; there is evidence that the sick, scary imagery of Halloween is also bad for children's minds.

That's because **young children are incapable of differentiating reality from illusion.** When they see a bloody zombie walking down the street, they think it's real, and they feel real fear.

Other bizarre holidays celebrated in America

That's why I think subjecting young children to the traditional Halloween routine is actually a form of **nutritional child abuse** (from the toxic candy) combined with damaging psychological episodes due to exposure to imagery of bloody humans and demonic creatures. This is all especially damaging to younger children. By the time children reach their teenage years, the ghoulish imagery is arguably less of a problem because they can now tell the difference between fact and fiction, but for small children these can be terrifying encounters.

Christmas seems like a healthier holiday. It's based on the principles of being good, sharing gifts and believing in flying reindeer that haul across the sky a fat man who engages in a global breaking-and-entering spree, trading gift-wrapped presents for milk and cookies. Okay, on second thought, that sounds more like somebody on a bad acid trip that somehow figured out a way to turn it into a commercial song (Rudolph the Red-Nosed Reindeer...).

Come to think of it, many holidays we celebrate seem to be based on bad acid trips or outright lies. Columbus Day, for example, is an outrageous celebration of a man who was guilty of the most heinous crimes against humanity thanks to the way he abused, tortured and murdered the American Indians he encountered in "the New World." (If you didn't know that, it's because actual history has been quietly removed from your public school history books...).

Easter is another truly bizarre acid trip holiday if there ever was one: since when did bunny rabbits lay eggs? And where did all the chocolate enter the scene, giving that cacao was practically unheard of in the Christian Biblical traditions from which the Easter holiday was largely derived? (Chocolate is from South America. Christianity is not).

Thanksgiving? Don't even get me started. It's not like the white man showed up in the New World and started *giving*. What they really did is more accurately described as "taking." Once the original British colonists had a stronghold in the east, they kept expanding westward, taking and taking until the Indians ended up on bone-dry desert lands, selling cigarettes and operating casinos. The holiday should be called "Thankstaking" - as in,

"Thanks for taking everything we had and leaving us with nothing to grow food on."

At least July 4th (Independence Day) sort of makes sense. The fireworks in the sky are supposed to remind people of the battles that were fought in order to win America's freedom from tyranny (British rule). But nobody seems to remember that anymore, so for most people July 4th has become just another excuse to eat ice cream and watch something exploding in the sky. Imagine Homer Simpson saying, "Woo-hoo! That was a big one!"

Presidents' Day is an interesting holiday. It celebrates the US government by shutting it down for one day. I agree that this is the best way to celebrate government. We should have this holiday more often.

But nothing takes the cake like Halloween - a bizarre and twisted celebration of maimed and bloodied humans, demons, witches, ghosts and other creatures of the night. Throw in a diarrhea-producing overdose of HFCS and cheap imitation chocolate candies and you've got a recipe for diabetes as well as steady future business for psychological counselors.

Try this experiment

If you really want to find out how bizarre Halloween is, just try this little trick in your neighborhood: this Thanksgiving, instead of erecting Christmas ornaments in your yard, string up all your Halloween decorations!

Have dead bodies strewn around your yard and trees, with demons and evil spirits peering out of your front windows. It's all standard fare on October 31st, of course, but for some reason this annoys the neighborhood when you do it one month later.

Make sure your acts of insanity fit in

This is how all the atrocities in human history have taken place. By the way, when people just go along with the insanities of everything else without questioning what's really happening around them, bad things tend to happen - like wars, or Nazi concentration camps.

The Holocaust was carried out by a bunch of people going along with the masses, doing what they were told and not having the presence of mind to ask if what they were doing made any real sense. (Yes, a few conscientious objectors knew what was going on and tried to stop it from the inside, but the masses just went right along as if killing fellow human beings was totally normal...).

That's why, personally, **I never throw dead bodies in my front yard,** no matter what day of the year it is. To me, it doesn't make any sense to celebrate the imagery of demons in darkness. Don't we have enough REAL beings of evil and darkness in our world the way it is right now? (Drug company executives, politicians, etc.). Do we really have to add to it with yet more dark imagery?

Only on Halloween do we see effigies of dead men hanging by a noose from a tree and somehow think, "Oh, that's okay, it's just for Halloween." I think such imagery is inappropriate every day of the year, **especially in the South,** for obvious historical reasons.

So if you have children, please think about healthier ways to celebrate various days of the year. Try to stick with more creative, positive imagery. Don't fall for the "dark side" of Halloween, and try to limit your child's exposure to candies, sweets and pastries. Although it's impossible to completely isolate them from such treats - and a very little treat every once in awhile won't cause permanent harm - don't allow them to drown themselves in processed sugar as so many do in the days following Halloween.

No wonder Halloween seems to celebrate **death** so much. If you eat all that candy every day of the year, you'll be dead before long.

The holiday commercialism agenda

You've got to wonder: If we have a national holiday that celebrates death, why don't we have a holiday that celebrates LIFE?

Truth be told, **all the holidays have been hijacked by corporations trying to sell more stuff.** Halloween, Easter and Valentine's Day are all about selling candy, sugar and junk food. Christmas is about "buying your way to joyousness" through gift-wrapped emptiness. It's sort of like the breast-cancer industries silly notion that "you can **cure** cancer by going shopping for more pink stuff." But, all in all, the holidays are an excuse to have you eat stuff not only to put you in a state of ill health, but also to keep you there. Truth be told, you can't find happiness - and you can't cure cancer - by buying more stuff.

I'm not trying to be especially cynical about all these holidays, by the way. I'm just thinking rationally about them, without the distortions of *blind tradition.* If you were a sentient being from an advanced civilization on another planet, and you came across planet earth on Halloween night in North America, what would you think of human civilization? I would think that maybe I had encountered some sort of bizarre indigenous race of superstitious beings engaged in some kind of tribal death tradition, and I would hurry up and snap some photos in hopes of getting them published in "National Galactic" magazine.

The headline story would be, "New race of humanoid tribal death worshippers discovered - exclusive photos inside'!"

Thank you, Mike, for allowing me to reprint your article.

To add more insult to injury there was an article that appeared in the NY Times that revealed some interesting things. It pointed out that the food industry is incapable of marketing healthier foods. That is not correct. They know precisely what they are doing. They sell the stuff that hooks your taste and keeps you coming back for more, despite the health ramifications to you. The article pointed out that the average American drinks 44.7 GALLONS of soda a year. One soda per day equals 12 extra pounds a year, what to speak of the potassium loss and the liver and kidney damage. Also, the Federal subsidies to the foods that keep you sick are around 80%. Yet, the subsidies for vegetables, fruits and grains are 3%.

Efforts to change the mindset toward a better diet have failed miserably. Why? It's because education takes a horrible back seat to the advertising dollars that push the worst foods on us. In 2009, the fast-food industry alone has spent more than $4 billion in marketing its crap to us. The benefit? The percentage of obese adults has doubled over the last 30 years and the percentage of obese kids has tripled. By 2018, health-related obesity costs are estimated to reach $344 billion.

In 2010, over 60 billion innocent animals and fish were slaughtered to satisfy the human tongue's desire for flesh and blood. Mankind goes on perpetrating these obscenities on defenseless creatures and yet they expect to find peace and happiness for themselves. Mahatma Gandhi said, "Protection of these innocent creatures means protection of the weak, the helpless, the dumb and the deaf. Man then becomes not the lord and master of all creation but its servant." The next step in the progress of human civilization has to be the liberation of the animals from the tyranny of mankind.

When around 10 million people are starving in the world today, most of the fertile land in the USA and other European countries is used to grow crops to feed animals, which in turn are consumed by human beings. This is an absolutely wasteful way of feeding ourselves. For every sixteen pounds of grains fed to cattle, only one pound of meat is produced. If there were a 10% reduction in meat production, there would be enough grain to feed 10 million people.

As you have read, most of the modern killer diseases are associated with the over-consumption of animal fats. As early as 1961, the Journal of the American Medical Association said that 90 – 97% of heart disease can be avoided by a vegetarian diet. Meat is suspected of causing a host of cancers such as cancer of the stomach, breast, bowels, blood and many others. Death by food poisoning is also an ever-present threat to flesh eaters. The high level of cholesterol in eggs means that they must be avoided completely if one wants to avoid heart disease. Nutritionally speaking, vegetables, fruits, nuts and grains are an excellent source of protein and calcium, and are easier to assimilate than that of flesh.

Former President Bill Clinton has adopted a vegan diet as well. In a short period of time he lost 24 pounds, his heart disease reversed, and he no longer is obsessed with the thought of premature death.

FEATURES OF MEAT_EATER	FEATURES OF PLANT_EATER	FEATURES OF HUMAN BEING
Licks and drinks	Sucks and drinks	Sucks and drinks
Sharp, pointed front teeth to tear flesh	No sharp, pointed teeth	No sharp, pointed teeth
Has claws	No claws	No claws
Intestinal tract only three times body length, so that rapidly decaying meat can pass out of body quickly	Intestinal tract 10-12 times body length. Fruits do not decay as rapidly as meat so can pass more slowly through body	Intestinal tract 10-12 times body length. Fruits do not decay as rapidly as meat so can pass more slowly through body
Small salivary glands in the mouth (not needed to pre-digest grains and fruits)	Well developed salivary glands, needed to pre-digest grains and fruits	Well developed salivary glands, needed to pre-digest grains and fruits
Acid saliva. No enzyme ptyalin to pre-digest grains	Alkaline saliva. Much ptyalin to pre-digest grains	Alkaline saliva. Much ptyalin to pre-digest grains
No flat back molar teeth to grind food	Flat back molar teeth to grind food	Flat back molar teeth to grind food
They can see during night	Cannot see during night	Cannot see during night
Can kill the prey without aid of weapons	Do not kill to eat	Cannot generally kill without the aid of weapon
They can digest raw meat easily	Do not eat meat	Cannot digest raw meat easily
Behavior is generally voracious	Behavior is not generally voracious	Becomes voracious by eating meat
Do not eat grass	Do not eat meat	Should not eat meat
No skin pores. Perspires through the tongue to cool body	Perspires through millions of skin pores	Perspires through millions of skin pores

It is extremely apparent that we have become a society of "Pimps, Hookers and Tricks." So, I will leave you with one final question: Do you really enjoy being a "Trick," repeatedly exploited by the "Pimps and Hookers?"

And what about the condition of the world we live in now. Mike Adams has put that subject very poignantly in another of his articles entitled, 'The Second American Revolution Has Begun'. What he had to say was this:

"There's a sense of desperation in America today. Their jobs are being exported out of the country, their health insurance is being dropped by employers, their dollars are becoming increasingly worthless with each passing day and their futures don't look very promising. They're angry, frustrated and desperate, so they take to the streets and protest. Occupy Wall Street! Occupy The Fed! Take to the streets!

"It's the right thing to do, but what most protestors – and nearly all Americans – don't fully grasp is that *nearly every powerful institution is a criminal racket*. It's not just Wall Street that's operated like a criminal mob, folks: it's the U.S. Congress. It's the health care industry. It's conventional agriculture, the mainstream media, the processed food manufactures, the government regulators [that were complicit with Monsanto in covering up the disastrous health effects of Roundup for the past thirty years] and of course the entire military industrial complex.

"Nearly everything around you is a criminal operation. The banks openly steal your homes while laundering money for global drug lords. The U.S. government runs illegal guns into Mexico while allowing cocaine and heroin back into the USA to be sold at pumped-up black market prices. The mainstream media broadcasts outright lies and complete fabrications as if they were fact. Much of modern medical "science" is complete quackery or fiction, funded by corporations for the purpose of expanding corporate power. The local water supply is intentionally contaminated with toxic poisons known as "fluoride" and the local food supply is tainted with other dangerous chemicals like aspartame, MSG and BPA.

"Your local hospital is almost certainly involved in a medical racket that seeks to insert high-profit medical procedure charges onto patient bills, and your local nursing home most likely throws granny in the hospital for a few days in order to get *triple billing* from Medicare upon her return. Doctors prescribe antibiotics because they get kickbacks from the drug companies, and the medical journals are little more than **science whores** who have been bought and paid for by the pharmaceutical industry. And don't forget vaccines, which have become the pathway through which infectious disease is actually *spread* among the population, using live viruses injected into innocent children. (http://www.naturalnews.com/033447_1...).

"**Wake the heck up, people!** Most of modern society is a giant con. Nearly every institution, every mega corporation, every government and nearly every politician or bureaucrat is really just a **criminal mobster** trying to steal your wealth or gain control over your actions and thoughts. Most institutions actually *cause* the very things they claim to be fighting against!

"The cancer industry actually *promotes* cancer, didn't you know? The DEA *runs drugs!* The ATF runs guns (http://www.naturalnews.com/032934_A...). The FDA keeps deadly drugs legal while trying to outlaw safe, affordable natural remedies.

"The EPA openly allows deadly toxic chemicals to be dumped into the environment (like mercury fillings from dental offices). The CDC actually promotes complete falsehoods about infectious disease in order to scare people into thinking everybody needs to get vaccinated. And then the vaccines are intentionally contaminated with live viruses in order to spread disease and make the CDC look even more important! (http://www. naturalnews.com/025760.html)

"Meanwhile the President is actively destroying the economic base of America, aided by feds who threaten businesses (like Gibson Guitars), which are only trying to manufacture quality American-made products. The purpose of all this? To destroy America's economy from the inside out. It is intentional. It is being *engineered.* The U.S. economy is *supposed* to collapse, by design. Get it?

"Beyond the economy alone, the entire "war on terror" is a complete and utter hoax, having been fabricated from the very start by government insiders. From 9/11 to present day terror, it has all been a pathetic and *cowardly* string of fabrications and staged events for the sole purpose of destroying freedom in America.

"Are you getting this? **Nearly everything you've been told is a lie.** Everything you hear on the mainstream news is either a complete fabrication or a wild distortion of reality. And the things you *don't* hear on the evening news are the things that really matter – things like the fact that your money is being quietly stolen from you by the Federal Reserve.

"Nearly everything you are told by the White House, or the EPA – or any government regulator – is a complete and total lie. There is no room for truth in a system of outright tyrannical lawbreaking. That's what we have today instead of government: a **cabal of criminal thugs** who operate with impunity while violating laws with complete disregard for human rights or the Bill of Rights.

"Did you know, for example, that the Obama administration runs a secret **death panel** that decides which Americans to add to a "kill list"? This kill list is then handed over to the President who decides which Americans to simply assassinate or murder. Think I'm making this up? Then why was it openly reported by Reuters? (http://www.naturalnews.com/033835_W...)

"Watch this astonishing interaction between ABC news reporter, Jake Trapper and White House Spokesperson Carney, who completely excuses the Obama administration's outright *murder* of an American citizen with absolutely zero evidence, no **due process,** no trial and no proper legal justification whatsoever. (http://www.naturalnews.tv/v.asp?v=1E3C8...)

"Do you wonder why so many people are sick and diseased today? Because the health care system is **designed to make you sick!**

"Do you wonder why so many people are bankrupt today? Because the financial system is **designed to keep you bankrupt!**

"Do you wonder why voters have so little power versus the corporations today? Because the political system is **designed to keep the corporation in power** while keeping you enslaved.

"Do you wonder why you are still paying $3 or $4 per gallon of gas? Because the energy industry is **designed to keep you enslaved to high-profit energy sources** while oppressing free energy technology.

"Do you ever wonder why **the best innovations in medicine, free energy and human consciousness are always suppressed?** Because the system is *designed* to destroy or censor any technologies that would lend themselves to longevity, freedom or increased awareness.

"Do you wonder why America remains in perpetual war with an unseen enemy? Because the whole system is **designed to operate in a state of perpetual warfare** so that the people can be kept in a state of constant fear while being denied their freedoms.

"This is why I invite you to **join the revolution** in whatever constructive way you can. Now is the time to make your voice heard, just like all those who are protesting right now.

"My only bit of wisdom to pass along in this regard is to **make sure it's your OWN** voice and don't let yourself be played by some organized globalist agenda that now wants to hijack the protests for their own nefarious purposes.

"The essence of freedom is **LIBERTY,** honest money, private property rights and a system of law that applies to *everyone.*

"YES, the globalist bankers are crooks. They probably deserve to be strung up in a public square somewhere, but even such actions should *never* be taken without *due process* and a proper trial. What's really wrong with

America today is that the criminal elements are running the show, from the White House to Wall Street. And it's time the people demanded that EVERYONE abide by the Constitution and the Bill of Rights. After all, didn't the President swear to protect it when he became President? So why does he now selectively ignore it?

"The revolution happening right now is a revolution born out of frustration, and although it seems to lack focus in the mixed messages heard on the street right now, it will soon coalesce into **a call for justice** and an end to the systems of tyranny that dominate the American landscape today.

The transition out of freedom and justice will be fraught with violence, I fear, and there will soon be martial law declared across our land. Be prepared for what's coming, and have no illusions that the second American Revolution is now at our doorstep. I only ask: What will you do with this opportunity? Will you stand for liberty and justice when it really counts?"

Thanks Mike. I could not have said it any better.

Last but not least, I have one final question to ask:

WHAT'S YOUR HEART'S CONDITION?

The question was not whether you had a "heart condition." It was specifically asking about your "heart's condition?" To put it another way, do you feel that you are soft hearted or hard hearted? By the time we are done with this, you will know one way or another.

Everyone says they are soft hearted and full of compassion. They have a pet dog or cat that they love to death, or some tropical fish or some type of bird. Yet, they have no problem eating the flesh of *other* creatures as long as they are not their pets. Does anyone see a bit of hypocrisy there? Maybe if they knew what the process was that put that flesh on their plate, they might have a different mindset.

Back in the 80's, the number of cattle "processed" in an hour was 50 to 175. Today it's up to 400 per hour at a given slaughterhouse.

Imagine an assembly line where men are standing shoulder to shoulder swinging knives and working at grinders at a frantic pace to make quota.

Do you think they are injured as well? Yes! And what about the men working the grinders? Do you think that maybe an arm or leg gets caught? Yes! Do you think they stop the grinder to free the limb and break the rhythm? Are you kidding me? So then, where does that limb go? Does it get processed along with the cows and wind up in your burger? Even if you can't prove that, do you really want to take the chance, especially since the USDA has allowed the companies themselves to do their own injury reporting?

Would it bother anyone to know that little chicks are run through a conveyor belt and dropped by the thousands onto a floor the size of two footballs fields where they can be fattened up in less than two months so you can eat them? What's even worse is that many of these chickens get sick or crippled and because of their numbers are left on the floor to be trampled by the others and still "processed" so they can be eaten as well?

What about the disease that comes with this "product," like salmonella, campylobacter, Chlamydia, tuberculosis, E.coli, staph, strep, botulism, worms, fowl typhoid, lice, mites and more? Then they are treated with enormous quantities of antibiotics, growth hormones, color enhancers, stink reducers and chemicals that emulate their natural smell, to make them appear bright, colorful, appetizing, healthy and tasty. Do you think that the sick creatures would be processed as well? Does a bear shit in the woods? Food poisoning anyone?

Seriously, do you really believe that the vibrant, red colored package of meat that you see in the supermarket is really that color? Understand that the nature of a dead body is to rot. As it is rotting or decomposing it starts to turn a grayish green, putrid looking color and starts to really smell. Well, that's where the wonders of science come in.

In New Jersey on Route 1, for example, there are chemical plants that work to fix that problem. With a dash of this and a drop of that, that putrid looking, foul smelling, rotting piece of flesh now has no odor and is a vibrant red and ready to go to the supermarket for you to buy.

What about what these *"food"* animals eat?

Well, cows have four stomachs because they are ruminants and need to process huge amounts of foods with cellulose content, like grass. Would it disturb you to know that the "Fraud and Drug Administration" allows them to eat dead pigs, horses and poultry? Mad Cow disease anyone? But the chickens are not vegetarians so they get treated to the dead, dying, diseased and decaying cows as their food. Yummmmy!

What if I barbeque?

Well, the fat from the flesh drips down onto the charcoals and releases a chemical called benzoapyrene, which is found in tobacco and which covers the flesh. When you eat it, it's the equivalent of smoking 300 cigarettes at one time. And what is the long-range effect of a flesh based diet? Cancer, heart disease, arthritis, etc..

Prescription drugs for life anyone?

This is why a flesh- and dairy-free, organic based vegan diet is not only the best and the healthiest diet to adhere to, but also the safest.

So, once again I ask, "What is your heart's condition? Soft or hard?" What you eat will answer that question.

References: *Fast Food Nation, Chew On This, EarthSave, University Of Mississippi School of Agriculture, National Cancer Institute, 2001*

Suffice it to say this is probably the heaviest waterhole you've ever been at. I've done my best to point you in the right direction but the rest is up to you. I certainly do hope that you can make a change for the better.

In retrospect, I sincerely wish I had all this knowledge before accepting the job with the butcher when I was young. In my early years, I was ignorant of the horrors wreaked on animals by the butchery of the meat industry and the horrors wreaked on humans as a result of consuming these products.

With what I know now, I could never have worked for a butcher and been a part of that animal and human holocaust. It is my sincere hope that this book will enlighten as many people as possible to not be as ignorant as I was and bring some sanity to the way we treat animals and the way we treat others and ourselves in this insane world.

For those of you that will attempt a transition, I suggest you start slowly. If your diet consists of mostly fast foods or flesh foods, at least one meal a day should be a large salad consisting of greens, like organic lettuce, kale and sprouts, cruciferous vegetable, like broccoli, bok choy, cabbage and onions, organic cucumbers, mushrooms, beans (garbanzo bean hummus makes a great salad dressing), nuts and seeds, and some berries. This one meal will provide you with incredible phytonutrients and antioxidents and can start you on the road to a complete change in building up your immune system. It all begins with the first bite.

Should you have any questions, feel free to contact me at anytime either at heshgoldstein@gmail.com or (808) 258-1177.

Aloha!

References: My thanks to Mike Adams, the "Health Ranger," for his permission in reprinting his article about '*What Halloween is Celebrating?*' And, '*The Second American Revolution Has Begun.*'

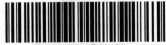

Made in the USA
Middletown, DE
20 July 2017